HEALTH & WEIGHT-LOSS BREAKTHROUGHS 2014

HEALTH&WEIGHT-LOSS
BREAKTHROUGHS 2014

FROM THE EDITORS OF Prevention®

RODALE®

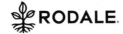

We inspire and enable people to improve their lives and the world around them.
For more of our products, visit **prevention.com** or call 800-848-4735.

CONTENTS

PART 3
Fitness Moves

PART 4
Nutrition News

PART 5
Mind Matters

PART 6
Beauty Breakthroughs

INTRODUCTION

The statistics aren't surprising: 75 percent of women use skin care products to look younger. More than half of Americans say they want to lose weight. Who doesn't want to look and feel great?

You hold the key to looking and feeling great in your hands. With the advice packed between the two covers of *Health & Weight-Loss Breakthroughs 2014*, you can take simple steps to look and feel terrific! We interviewed the top experts, read the medical journals, tested the products, tried out the exercises, and tasted the recipes to ensure that this book is filled with simple solutions to help you. We searched for the newest health breakthroughs on weight loss, nutrition, fitness, mind matters, and beauty. And we offer simple ways to apply these medical breakthroughs to your own life.

In Part 1: Health Breakthroughs, you'll discover "12 Steps to Living Longer and Stronger." Read how to protect yourself against two all-too-common conditions: osteoporosis and back pain. You'll learn how to boost your immunity and keep your family safe from foodborne illnesses.

Are you struggling with your weight? In Part 2: Weight-Loss Wisdom, you'll find out why. Then you'll learn how to love your belly—at any age and bust some pervasive weight-loss myths, including "The Truth about Sugar." Next give yoga a try—for your health and happiness.

Turn to our Bonus Weight-Loss Cookbook for this year's best *Prevention* recipes. They're delicious, nutritious, and easy to make. Our favorites include the Pumpkin-Bacon Pancakes, Pear Toddy, Sausage-Stuffed Mushrooms, Grilled Chicken with Mango Mojo, Mango-Shrimp Rice Noodles, Pistachio Clouds with Fresh Fruit, and Baked Maple Pears.

We hope you feel inspired to get up off the couch and exercise with Part 3: Fitness Moves. Try our "Superfast Indoor Workout" when the weather's not cooperating and our "Walking Workout" when it is. Find some great gift ideas to boost the health of everyone on your gift list.

Then in Part 4: Nutrition News, you'll learn how to eat to live, rather than live to eat. Who wouldn't want to know "What Doctors Really Eat." We then focus on two superfoods: greens and foods with probiotics. As a bonus, you'll read about "Foods That Fight Pain."

Are you too pooped to pop? Stressed? Fried? Check out the new strategies and innovations in Part 5: Mind Matters. You'll find "2-Minute Stress Solutions" and learn how to "Sleep Like a Baby Tonight."

You'll look as good as you'll feel after following the tips in Part 6: Beauty Breakthroughs. Eat better to look better with our "Beauty Foods." Make the most of a rainbow of colors with "Color Therapy." And then protect your body's largest organ, your skin, with our chapter on "Sun Safety."

We've filled *Health & Weight-Loss Breakthroughs 2014* with the newest and best health and weight-loss news and information. Here's to your health and happiness!

Part 1

HEALTH
BREAKTHROUGHS

CHAPTER 1

12 STEPS TO LIVING LONGER AND STRONGER

Dr. Sanjay Gupta advises millions on TV about medical breakthroughs and healthier habits. But he— and his family—also take these lessons to heart. Here are his 12 steps to living longer and stronger.

There are places in this world where heart disease is almost unknown—and Sanjay Gupta, MD, chief medical correspondent for CNN, has studied them carefully for clues to their success. They're not necessarily the societies with the most advanced medicine. In fact, Western medical care has barely made inroads among some of these people, including Papua New Guineans and Mexico's Tarahumara Indians. Their secret? They're not sedentary. Even more important, they eat whole foods. And they consume very little sugar—"pretty much once a year, when fruit ripens," Dr. Gupta says.

Dr. Gupta has logged some serious hours exploring the science behind all this—not just for heart health, but for brain health and cancer reduction too. He has traveled to Okinawa to meet with 100 year olds. He has personally tested the health benefits of meditation. And each step of the way, he has incorporated the lessons he has learned into his own lifestyle. The result? He's incredibly fit, especially for someone with such demands on his time—as a TV correspondent, a practicing neurosurgeon, the author of three books (including his medical novel, *Monday Mornings*), and a husband and father of three young girls. In his own words, here's how he does it—and how you can too.

DON'T THINK OF EXERCISE AS OPTIONAL

The president of CNN Worldwide is Jim Walton. If he says, "I need to meet with you," I'm going to meet with him. That's a huge priority for me. But my well-being and fitness are also huge priorities for me, so I give them the same degree of importance. If you have a busy day, the inclination is to let exercise fall off the radar, but the meeting with the boss will not. I treat exercise like a meeting with the boss.

PUMP YOUR HEART TO BETTER YOUR BRAIN

Over the past 3 years, I've gotten involved in triathlons, which include swimming, biking, and running. Aerobic exercise increases cardiac output, meaning the heart's pumping capacity. But even more interesting is new research showing that patients with better cardiac output also have larger brains, with more neural growth factors and even some new cells. It's a brain that's more efficient.

MOVE IT OR LOSE IT

Incorporating movement into your everyday life is probably even better for you than going to the gym. From an evolutionary standpoint, humans are designed to move, not to sit or lie down for 23 hours a day and exercise for one. For people with desk jobs, this can be tough. I've got a pullup bar hanging above the door in my office. I don't do a lot of weights, but I do push-pull exercises—pushups, pullups, situps, using my own body weight—that I can do on the road when I travel. Strength training and isometrics seem to be particularly good for decreasing body mass index and increasing HDL ['good' cholesterol].

I also keep a jump rope in my office. One of our producers doesn't have a chair at his desk, so he stands. Other people sit on those big exercise balls.

Something else we now do at both the office and the hospital is walking meetings. If we have to meet, we'll walk. I find the meetings are much more productive. I don't know why. Maybe it's because our brains are getting bigger simultaneously.

GET YOUR KIDS IN THE ACT

Before I started training for triathlons, I had to talk to my wife [lawyer Rebecca Gupta] about the fact that I might spend 4 hours on a Saturday morning exercising. That's potentially 4 hours away from our kids. So now we have jogging strollers. We have a Burley child trailer for the back of the bike, so I can take a kid and let her nap in the Burley. I'll take the older kids to the park, while I swim in the lake.

STOP EATING BEFORE YOU'RE FULL

In Japan, I interviewed a woman who was 103 years old and still selling oranges. I asked her how she stayed young. She said she dated younger men, which I thought was funny. But there was a lot more to her story than that. Something I learned in Okinawa was the concept of hara hachi bu. You push the plate away when you're 80 percent full. It made sense to me from a neuroscience perspective because it takes 15 to 20 minutes for your brain to register that you're in fact full.

"Push the plate away when you're 80 percent full."

FALL OUT OF LOVE WITH SUGAR

My wife and I do not keep sweets in the house. When our kids go to birthday parties, they scrape the frosting off the cake because it tastes too sweet to them. People think the problem with sugar is that it makes you fat. But it's not just inches around your waist. Sugar is a potential toxin. The liver becomes fatty, and it starts to release small, dense particles of LDL, which are the most damaging kind for blood vessels. There is also some interesting new data suggesting that a third of some common cancers, including breast and colon cancer, have insulin receptors on them, so you could be fueling indolent cancers. Ice cream is my weakness. But I've got to walk to get it. The store is more than a mile away. I'll walk there with the girls once a month.

GROW A GARDEN

I will candidly tell you that as a medical student, I never had any nutritional training, which is crazy. Most of what I've learned has been on my own. And it's not only the science that's important, but learning how to make it work with my wife and kids. We're primarily vegetarian. We also have a little kitchen garden. The kids love that, and we feel it teaches them that food comes from the ground as opposed to a store.

We don't keep meat at home, but we might order a small portion when we go out. Most steak houses have the petit fillet. Historically, people didn't eat meat that often. And when they did, it was after chasing a woolly mammoth.

EAT A RAINBOW DIET

I made a list of the nutrients that people would like to get in a supplement and found I could get them all by eating seven colorful foods a day. I mix it up as much as possible between vegetables, fruits, and nuts: red, orange, yellow, green, blue, purple, some brown. That gives me all the vitamins, minerals, and antioxidants I need. So when it comes to supplements, I take omega-3 fatty acids, and that's all. I don't take a multivitamin. I don't take the "broccoli in a pill." By the way, broccoli and kale are powerhouses for protein, which I bring up only because people say, "You're not eating meat. Are you getting enough protein?"

DON'T SKIMP ON SLEEP

Bill Clinton was famous for talking about how little sleep he got, and it was seen as a badge of honor. It was the same for us in the medical profession until studies started showing that you're putting your heart at risk by not getting adequate sleep. You can increase your levels of cortisol, a stress hormone, and this probably increases your blood pressure and makes your arteries stiffer and less elastic too. And the data on how much less effective you are at work the next day are pretty good.

STOP MEDICATING, START MEDITATING

What's the saying, "In God we trust—everyone else bring data"? I wanted to know that if I meditated, it would make a difference. I have a history of heart disease in my family. My father had bypass surgery in his early fifties. I'm not a very high-stress person. But Herbert Benson [MD, of the Mind/Body Medical Institute in Massachusetts] took video of me when I meditated. He showed me

"Over the past 3 years, I've gotten younger from a biological perspective."

the different muscles in my face and how they relaxed. He measured my blood pressure and heart rate, and they came down. The key for me was learning to clear my mind. Herbert taught me to focus on a specific word for 5 minutes, followed by 10 minutes of classic meditation—for a total of 15 minutes. It's pretty powerful. After I meditate, I feel great. The same thing that would have annoyed me 20 minutes earlier doesn't bother me at all 20 minutes later.

SCHEDULE "YOU" TIME

I'm pretty busy. I do rounds in the hospital early in the morning. I do the morning shows on TV a lot. Every Monday I perform surgery. That actually seems

ADD 2 YEARS TO YOUR LIFE IN 10 MINUTES

You already know that getting 30 minutes of aerobic activity at least five times a week has major health benefits. Now, new research shows that tallying up that much—or even less—regular exercise might extend your life.

In a large study, National Cancer Institute researchers found that people with a high activity level, about what you'd get from walking briskly for an hour daily, lived 4.5 years longer than their more sedentary peers. Before you roll your eyes about anyone who has an extra hour a day, get this: Those who had a low activity level, equal to walking 75 minutes a week—just over 10 minutes daily—lived almost 2 years longer than nonexercisers. Extra pounds weren't a factor; people of all weights reaped similar benefits. What matters is making time to exercise.

The study didn't look at incidental activities such as housecleaning or running errands. It focused on leisure-time workouts, such as walking or playing sports.

"If you want to live longer, any physical activity is good," says Steven Moore, PhD, the study's lead author. "But more is better."

pretty relaxing to me now, after doing it for 20 years. But I'm working on so many things simultaneously: documentaries, breaking news, publicity for my new book. One survival method for me is taking my calendar and putting "Sanjay time" on it. I spend part of that period meditating, but I also spend part of it reflecting on things. I'll make lists of everything I'm supposed to do rather than trying to remember it all. Today there were two of these 30-minute periods on my calendar. I don't know if it makes me more efficient, but it makes me feel in control, so I feel better about things.

GROW YOUNGER—YES, YOU CAN!

You want to live your life like an incandescent light bulb—not a fluorescent bulb that flickers at the end, but one that burns brightly and then suddenly goes out. And I think diet and exercise as I've outlined really help.

But the flip side of that is you can make yourself younger. Over the past 3 years, since I've been doing triathlons, I've gotten younger from a biological perspective. One way to measure biological age is to look at your telomeres—the little strands of genetic material at the end of chromosomes. They get shorter as you grow older. But we've recently learned that they can shorten at a slower rate or even stop shortening. I had my telomeres measured for a story I was working on 7 years ago, and I had them measured again last year. My telomeres were actually longer the second time.

CHAPTER 2

KITCHEN CHECKUP

Is your kitchen making you sick? It very well could be. According to the Centers for Disease Control and Prevention, 1 in 6 Americans, about 48 million people, get sick from foodborne illness each year.

Most of us like to think we know the basics of kitchen cleanliness, whether it's how to handle raw chicken or that veggies should be thoroughly washed before eating. But restaurant kitchens are held to much more exacting standards than most of us ever impose on ourselves.

We decided to see what we could all learn, so we sent a kitchen-cleanliness expert, Mark Nealon, to scrutinize the kitchens of two *Prevention* families as they prepared dinner on a busy weeknight. A former New York City restaurant inspector, Nealon now helps restaurants institute the very best food safety practices to avoid being slapped with health-code violations. These two moms, both of whom consider themselves quite safety conscious, were shocked—as you'll be—to discover where their kitchen habits fell short.

CASE STUDY #1

Food preparation is often a hectic family affair for Stacey, a literary agent; her husband, Jeremy Zirin, an equity strategist; and their daughters—Samantha, Alea, and identical twins Chelsea and Talia —in Haworth, New Jersey. All six of them crowd into the kitchen to help out. Under Nealon's watchful eye, Stacey and her family put together a quick pizza, using premade crust from the supermarket, and a salad.

Stacey says that she tries to avoid obvious food safety mistakes, such as letting her kids share eating utensils. But she adds, "I don't have time to sanitize everything, and I know I'm probably overlooking some dangers."

Her biggest worry is the state of her two jam-packed refrigerators. She keeps one in a nearby closet to accommodate all the food she buys.

"I know I overbuy food, and things get forgotten until they're moldy," Stacey says. "Then I worry about bacteria from spoiled food contaminating the other food we'll be eating."

What Stacey Is Doing Right

She keeps the dog out of the kitchen. Oliver, a Shih Tzu, is not allowed in during meal prep and dining, mostly to keep him out of the way.

The inspector's advice: "This is actually an important safety measure," says Nealon, who has a dog himself. "Petting an animal or feeding him scraps could contaminate your hands with dangerous germs." And never let cats jump up on your counter. Their paws carry lots of bacteria, which you want to keep off your work surface. In fact, keep cats away from all food-preparation areas.

She uses plastic containers for storage of dried foods such as rice and cereal. This keeps critters out of foods.

The inspector's advice: To avoid chemicals leaching into foods, be sure containers are made of food-grade plastic. Look for those bearing a seal from NSF International, which is a safety certification organization.

She keeps her kitchen sponge upright in a holder. This allows it to dry completely between uses, Nealon says, whereas damp sponges breed bacteria.

The inspector's advice: At the very least, wash sponges with antibacterial soap after use and wring out well. You can also sanitize a sponge by microwaving it for 30 seconds or running it through the dishwasher. No matter what method you use, make sure the sponge air-dries completely.

What Stacey Is Doing Wrong

Her fridges are too warm. When Nealon measured the temperature in both the kitchen fridge and the second one, they were 52° and 53°F—dangerously high! "Your fridge should be set at 40°F or below," he says. "Above that, bacteria start to grow, and you risk serious sickness."

The inspector's advice: Buy a digital refrigerator thermometer and check it often.

Her fridge is overloaded. In fact, both refrigerators were jammed full, which prevents proper air circulation and cooling and can hasten food spoilage.

The inspector's advice: Leave more space between items. Less crowding will also help prevent food from being pushed to the back and forgotten. Crowding of items does not affect the freezer, however. In fact, a full freezer cools more efficiently.

She keeps food too long. After a sniff to check for spoilage, Stacey was going

QUICK QUIZ

How kitchen safety savvy are you? Take our quiz and then see the answers on page 14.

1. Is 45°F cold enough for your fridge?
2. Is it okay to sip from a bottle or cup and save leftovers?
3. The homemade label on a food says "bean dip." Good enough?
4. Is a packed-full fridge jammed too tight?
5. Is it okay to store meat and poultry on a middle fridge shelf?
6. Should frozen chicken sit out to thaw?
7. Home-canned food is a good, healthy option, right?
8. Is a packed-full freezer stuffed too full?
9. Is a plastic or wood cutting board better?
10. Are pets allowed in the kitchen?
11. Should you wipe up with a cloth or paper towel?

to top her pizza with fried eggplant slices she'd bought a week and a half before. "But just because something still smells fine doesn't mean it's safe to eat," says Nealon.

The inspector's advice: Toss the eggplant; as a general rule, cooked vegetables aren't good after 3 to 4 days. "Remember that your fridge doesn't stop the growth of pathogens; it just slows it down," he says. Date food before refrigerating. If you have any doubts about freshness, don't eat it.

She stores food that could be tainted. Stacey's kids love to scatter cheese on the pizza—and eat some from the bag, which transfers bacteria from their fingers to the contents. When the bag goes back in the fridge, bacteria multiply and could make them sick the next time they eat the cheese.

The inspector's advice: Place some mozzarella into a bowl for the kids, and toss what remains.

QUICK ANSWERS

Here are the answers to the Quick Quiz on page 13. How does your kitchen measure up?

1. No. 40°F is the max.
2. Never. Remaining beverage could be tainted.
3. Nope. You also need to date it.
4. Yes. Food needs room for cold air to circulate.
5. No. Meat should be stored on the bottom shelf.
6. No way. Bacteria can grow before it's fully defrosted.
7. Not unless you canned it yourself and know it was properly done.
8. No. A full freezer actually cools more efficiently.
9. Either is fine. More important than the material is cleaning the board thoroughly between uses.
10. No, and certainly not on the counters. If you pet your dog when cooking, food can be contaminated.
11. Paper. Cloth towels might be germy.

COMMUTER CONCERN

The scariest part about commuting isn't the traffic: Your trip to the office could make you sick.

What's the first thing you do when you get to work? If it's answer e-mails or scarf down a quick breakfast at your desk, you might want to put washing your hands at the top of your to-do list. Gas pump handles, escalator rails, and many other things that you commonly come in contact with on your commute are germy enough to make you sick, according to new research by the hygiene products and services company Kimberly-Clark Professional.

Testers swabbed high-trafficked surfaces in six major US cities, measuring for levels of adenosine triphosphate (ATP). ATP exists in all bacteria, including staphylococcus and E. coli, and its presence is a good indication that something is unsanitary.

"Surfaces with ATP readings of 300 or higher could make you ill," says study coauthor Kelly Arehart, PhD.

CASE STUDY #2

Kathleen Egan, a science teacher, and her husband, Richard Egan, a police officer, of Valley Stream, New York, take food safety seriously.

"Richard will clean up immediately after we eat; sometimes while we eat," laughs Kathleen, who at the time of the inspection was pregnant with the couple's second child. On the other hand, Kathleen confesses to sometimes letting her daughter eat a morsel that's fallen to the floor.

"I've heard it's okay if it's within 5 seconds. Is that true?" she asks.

"It is usually safe to follow the so-called 5-second rule," says Nealon. "Bacteria haven't had a chance to grow. But don't wait longer than that, or put the food back in the fridge."

That aside, it didn't take Nealon long to discover some serious mistakes the Egans were making while they prepared pasta, chicken, and salad.

WARNING: MOBILE MENACE

One in six cell phones is contaminated with fecal matter due to poor hand-washing habits, according to research from the University of London. To stay healthy, use gadget-friendly antibacterial towelettes, such as Wireless Wipes ($3; wirelesswipes.com).

Here are the percent of common surfaces that are dangerously dirty. Avoid touching them when possible, and use hand sanitizer when you can't.

71 percent of gas pump handles

68 percent of sidewalk mailbox handles

43 percent of escalator rails

41 percent of ATM buttons

40 percent of parking meters

35 percent of crosswalk buttons

35 percent of vending machine buttons

What Kathleen Is Doing Right

She washes her hands for a full 20 seconds before handling food. This is key to preventing contamination.

The inspector's advice: Work up a lather with antibacterial soap, get under your fingernails, and then dry your hands with paper towels—not a dirty dish towel that might have been used to wipe up food spills.

She defrosts chicken in the fridge. Thawing poultry, meat, or fish in the fridge is the safest bet.

The inspector's advice: If you need to defrost more quickly, do it in the microwave or under cold running water in the sink. Never leave a partially frozen protein food to thaw on the counter, where it can grow bacteria by the time it's completely defrosted.

She uses a fresh spoon to serve cooked chicken. A spoon that has touched raw poultry could contaminate the food with salmonella.

The inspector's advice: Even rinsing a spoon under hot water won't kill germs, so keep clean ones on hand for serving.

What Kathleen Is Doing Wrong

She defrosts on the top fridge shelf. No matter how well wrapped, raw poultry, meat, or fish can easily leak juices and contaminate foods below.

The inspector's advice: Always defrost and store raw protein foods on the lowest shelf in your fridge.

She hand-washes her plastic cutting board. Immediately after slicing the chicken, germaphobe Richard scrubbed the board with hot water and soap before chopping vegetables on it. But that's not enough.

The inspector's advice: Cutting boards need to be sanitized by having boiling water poured over them or being run through the dishwasher. This should be done even after cutting vegetables, which have been linked with salmonella outbreaks.

She serves her family home-canned tomato sauce. Kathleen wanted to top her pasta with a jar of sauce a friend had canned. But home-canned goods—even from a farm stand—can be tainted with botulism, despite looking and smelling fine.

The inspector's advice: Realize that cooking does not destroy botulism. Never eat food you haven't canned properly yourself—especially if the seal doesn't pop audibly when you open the jar.

60 SECONDS TO SAFER FOOD

A sink and a microwave are surprisingly good weapons in the war against food poisoning, according to new research published in the journal *Food Control*. Jalapeños contaminated with salmonella that were quickly dunked in water, then microwaved for 25 seconds and cooled in clean water, were fresh tasting and safe to eat.

She stores half-full sippy cups in the fridge. Once the germs from a child's mouth are in the liquid, they will multiply—even in the fridge—and could make her sick when she drinks again.

The inspector's advice: Dump leftover liquids and start fresh.

SAFER GRILLING

Now that your kitchen is inspection ready, what about when you take it outdoors to barbecue? Here's how to extend your safety net to the great outdoors.

START WITH A SOAK. Marinating meat in a mix of vinegar (or lemon juice), fresh herbs, and garlic adds flavor and helps prevent the formation of carcinogens called heterocyclic amines. If the mixture contains oil, be sure to let the excess drip off the meat (or pat it dry with a paper towel) to avoid flare-ups.

GET FINICKY ABOUT FAT. Before grilling meat and poultry, take the time to trim any excess fat. The smoke caused by fat dripping onto the hot grill contains other harmful chemicals called polycyclic aromatic hydrocarbons. And don't press down on your burgers. You want to keep the juices in the patties, not in the flames.

AVOID OVERCOOKING. Don't char your meat. Scraping off burned parts won't get rid of the offending compounds. A few light grill marks are fine. Don't go further than that.

CLEAN THE GRATE. A dirty grill is unsightly, and it's also unhealthy. You wouldn't want those charred bits to hitch a ride on your next meal. Clean the grate after you finish cooking (while the grill is still hot but not turned on), using a long-handled, steel-bristled brush.

MAKE A SAFER SALAD. The raw egg recipes, such as Caesar Salad, can be back on your menu without fear of salmonella, thanks to a new hot-water bath that kills bacteria without cooking the eggs. Look for Safest Choice, the largest national brand. Expect to pay about $4 per dozen.

HOW THE INSPECTOR KEEPS HIS KITCHEN CLEAN

Food-safety expert Mark Nealon suggests you do what he does in his own home.

SANITIZE WITH HEAT. When Nealon uses tongs to put raw poultry or meat on the grill, he also places the tips on the grill. He then closes the lid, leaving the handles outside. The intense heat zaps bacteria, so he can safely use the same tongs to remove the cooked food.

WASH BEFORE YOU CUT. People usually don't wash fruits such as melons before cutting into them. But such produce grows in dirt, and your knife can easily transfer pathogens—such as the deadly Listeria that recently contaminated cantaloupes—from the rind to the flesh. So avoid buying precut produce, and give all fruits and vegetables a thorough cleansing with a produce brush before slicing. Even better: Place vinegar in a spray bottle and give your produce a spritz. Wait 30 seconds, and then rinse thoroughly.

PUT COOKED FOOD AWAY PROMPTLY. Never contaminate food with your hands or utensils that have been in your mouth. And refrigerate it within 2 hours after cooking—otherwise, toss it.

SANITIZE WITH BOILING WATER. Before he cooks, Nealon puts a pot of water on the stove. That way, it's ready to purge germs from utensils and sponges before and after he uses them. When he's done, he dumps the water in the sink to clean it as well.

CHAPTER 3

INNER STRENGTH

Half of all women over 50 will break a bone. But it's never too late to prevent frightening fractures. The following smart, simple steps can help you—and your skeleton—stay strong and healthy for life.

Nobody expects to break a bone. As we race through our happily hectic days, we take for granted the 206 bones in our skeletons. But when one snaps, everything changes. A break might mean doctors' appointments, x-rays, a cast, or even surgery, physical therapy, and months of limited mobility. And if you're over 40, you might also worry that this fracture will be just the first of many to come.

What you fear is osteoporosis, the disease that leaves bones brittle and prone to fractures. It often occurs in the first few years after menopause, when bone loss accelerates due to dropping estrogen levels. A matrix of minerals, bone is constantly broken down and rebuilt by the body at a microscopic level: If the breakdown consistently exceeds the buildup, bones lose density.

Eight million women and 2 million men age 50 and older have osteoporosis, and some 34 million more Americans have osteopenia, a stage of bone decline that occurs before full-blown osteoporosis.

But even in midlife and beyond, women can still prevent bone disease. Here is our *Prevention* bone-protection plan.

STAY STRONGER LONGER

The most effective way to protect your bones is to make sure that you're getting enough calcium, vitamin D, and protein, whether it's through food or with the help of supplements. Even though you reach your bone-building peak around age 30, getting the right amounts of these key nutrients throughout your life is crucial to keeping your skeleton healthy. Here's the latest expert advice on where to start.

Calcium

What you need: 1,000 milligrams a day for women ages 19 to 50; 1,200 milligrams for those over 50, per the Institute of Medicine (IOM). This mineral is the single most important component in building and maintaining healthy bone density.

Where to get it: Dairy products—especially fat-free or low-fat milk and yogurt—are excellent sources, and they account for about 72 percent of Americans' calcium intake. (If you're lactose intolerant, lactose-free products provide calcium too.) Other great sources include canned sardines and salmon, calcium-fortified orange juice and dry breakfast cereals, Cheddar cheese, and tofu (if prepared with calcium sulfate). (Check out the calcium content of various foods at prevention.com/calcium-food.)

Supplemental sources: Your body can handle only about 500 to 600 milligrams of calcium in one 6- to 8-hour period and absorbs only about 30 percent of that. If you consume only 1 to 2 cups of milk and/or yogurt daily, you'll come closer to meeting your daily requirements if you also take a daily supplement that provides 500 milligrams of calcium citrate or 600 milligrams of calcium carbonate, according to Ethel Siris, MD, director of the osteoporosis clinic at Columbia University Medical Center in New York City. (It's okay if your dose is included in your daily multivitamin.) Calcium carbonate should be taken with meals for best absorption, but calcium citrate can be taken at any time of day.

Can you take too much? While it's not a common problem, the IOM warns against consuming too much calcium. At elevated levels, the mineral can cause kidney stones, and it was linked in one major study to a slightly heightened risk of heart attack. It's not connected, however, with the "calcifications" that might turn up on mammograms. The IOM sets the upper limit of safety for women over 50 at 2,000 milligrams of calcium a day.

Vitamin D

What you need: 600 IU daily for people ages 1 to 70; 800 IU above age 70, according to the IOM.

Where to get it: You can't absorb calcium without vitamin D, which can sometimes be found in the same sources, such as dairy products (a glass of vitamin D–fortified milk has about 120 IU). Additionally, it's in fatty fish such as salmon and mackerel, egg yolks, and D–fortified breakfast cereals. Vitamin D is also synthesized by the skin when sunlight touches it, but if you use sunscreen, have very dark skin, or live in a cloudy climate, you might be limited in how much your body can manufacture.

Supplemental sources: A blood test can confirm if you're getting enough D. If you need more, Dr. Siris recommends a supplement with 400 IU of vitamin D (as cholecalciferol).

Can you take too much? The IOM also sets an upper limit (4,000 IU daily) for vitamin D, but it's best to stay well under that. Unless you're diagnosed with a severe deficiency, avoid supplements greater than 1,000 units a day.

NOT FOR WOMEN ONLY

While osteoporosis is often thought of as a women's illness, men aren't immune. Their bone loss is more gradual than women's, because they don't undergo menopause, but up to one out of every four men over age 50 will break a bone due to osteoporosis—making it more prevalent than prostate cancer.

The outlook for men after such a fracture is worse than it is for women: Men are more likely to die within a year after breaking a hip than are women.

Protein

What you need: Up to 77 grams a day for a woman who weighs about 154 pounds, according to a 2010 multiuniversity study published in *Aging Health*. While the RDA for a woman of this weight is 56 grams, the research suggests that another 21 grams a day can improve bone strength. When you increase dietary protein, you increase calcium absorption and a natural growth factor called IGF-1, which is important for bone formation.

   Where to get it: Poultry, lean meats, fish, beans, tofu, and fat-free or low-fat dairy products all pack protein. For a sense of how much: Three ounces of cooked beef has about 28 grams of protein, 3 ounces of sardines has 21 grams, a cup of lentils has 18 grams, and a cup of yogurt has 14 grams.

BONE-BUILDING MOVES

One way to strengthen your skeleton is with exercise. Why? "Exercise stimulates bone formation, because bone put under moderate stress responds by building density, and, depending on your age and workout regimen, it can either increase or maintain bone-mass density," says Steven Hawkins, PhD, professor of exercise science at California Lutheran University. That's why physical activity can reduce your risk of sustaining a hip fracture, which is usually caused by osteoporosis, by as much as a whopping 50 percent.

   Dr. Hawkins cautions that if you already have osteoporosis or osteopenia, your best option is to protect your bones by improving stamina and balance, which will help you avoid falls. He recommends cardiovascular-endurance exercise such as walking, low-impact aerobics, and dancing. These will serve the additional purpose of building muscle strength, which will help keep you

Protein: 3 ounces of fish can pack in a full 21 grams of protein.

Calcium: Tofu prepared with calcium sulfate is a good nondairy source of the mineral.

Vitamin D: An egg yolk contains 10 percent of your daily vitamin D.

upright and free from fracture-inducing falls. (Consult a health professional before undertaking any regimen, of course.)

If your bones are still healthy, working out with weight-training machines, free weights, or resistance bands, as well as doing exercises that use your body weight as resistance (situps and pushups, for example), will all build your bone density. The single best way to increase bone density is jumping (think jumping rope, jump squats, plyometrics), according to Dr. Hawkins.

To build bone mass in the three areas most prone to breakage from falls—the spine, hips, and forearms—Dr. Hawkins suggests this trio of moves: biceps curls, triceps extensions, and Romanian dead lifts. For instructions on how to do them, visit prevention.com/boneexercises.

YOUR DENSITY DESTINY

The gold standard for assessing bone health is a test called DXA (for dual-energy x-ray absorptiometry). The completely painless 10-minute scan typically measures bone-mineral density in the hip and lower spine.

Many women can wait until 65 to have the procedure, according to Sundeep Khosla, MD, a bone specialist at the Mayo Clinic in Rochester, Minnesota, and there's no need for most women to get a baseline test prior to menopause, he says. But if you're at high risk, you should get the test sooner—within 3 years of menopause, at the latest.

The scoring for the test is based on the average bone density of a 30-year-old woman, whose T-score, as it's called, is zero. If your T-score falls between -1 and -2.5, your diagnosis will be osteopenia, which you should take as a wake-up call to do all you can to preserve your bones and try to prevent the development of osteoporosis. If your score is -2.6 or lower, you're considered to have full-blown osteoporosis.

Are you at risk? Everyone's odds of osteoporosis increase with age: The older you get, the more likely you are to develop the disease. But many other factors can also affect your chances—and some of them are within your power to change. Here are some of the most common contributors to osteoporosis risk.

• You have a family history of osteoporosis among men or women on either side.

• You've already had a low-impact fracture, which is a break caused by only a mild trauma.

• You were treated for at least 3 months at any point in your life with oral steroids, which weaken bones.

• You've got a bone-robbing disease such as rheumatoid arthritis.

• You had an early or abrupt menopause, which can result from chemotherapy or removal of ovaries, lowering your estrogen levels.

• You consume too much caffeine (more than 375 milligrams or about 4 cups of coffee a day), salt (more than 2,300 milligrams daily), or alcohol (more than one drink for women per day; more than two per day for men).

• You smoke.

FIVE SUPPLEMENTS NOT TO OVERDO

Don't assume more is better. Many supplements and multivitamins contain two to 10 times some RDAs. Such high doses, combined with the nutrients you get from food, can tip you over the maximum and lead to health issues such as kidney stones and liver damage. Belowe are the most common culprits:

NUTRIENT	RDA	MAX AMOUNT
Vitamin A	700 micrograms	3,000 micrograms
Vitamin D	600 IU	4,000 IU
Vitamin E	22.4 IU	4,000 IU
Calcium	1,000–1,200 milligrams	2,000 milligrams
Iron	18 milligrams for women under 50; 8 milligrams for women 50 and over	45 milligrams

If you're not sure how much at risk you are, the World Health Organization has devised a free online test called FRAX. By answering a few simple questions, you can determine your chances (given as a percentage) of suffering an osteoporotic fracture in the next 10 years. You can find the FRAX calculator at shef.ac.uk/frax.

BONE PROTECTION IN A PILL?

If you're diagnosed with osteoporosis, your doctor might advise pharmaceutical help, likely from a class of drugs called bisphosphonates, which are approved by the FDA to help strengthen bone. Now the most frequently prescribed medications for osteoporosis, members of this class include Fosamax, Boniva, Actonel, and Reclast.

Bisphosphonates work by slowing down the rate at which the body breaks down and builds up bone, the idea being that this helps the bones retain calcium and thus density.

"Used properly, these drugs are generally effective and safe at preserving bone mass," says Felicia Cosman, MD, senior clinical director of the National Osteoporosis Foundation.

However, you should be aware of a rare complication of using bisphosphonates long term (7 years or more): a distinctive type of fracture of the thighbone, which is usually one of the strongest bones in the body. Called an atypical femur fracture, this side effect is rare, but because millions of women have been taking these drugs, thousands could be at risk of these fractures. Researchers are still trying to understand who is most susceptible. These fractures are often signaled by pain in the area of the thigh or groin. If you take bisphosphonates and have a new or worsening pain of this kind, you should contact your doctor right away.

Additionally, if you take bisphosphonates, you should talk to your doctor at least once a year to make sure the benefits of continuing the medication outweigh the risks. Doctors today generally don't prescribe the drugs for longer than 5 years, though in some cases, patients might be able to resume taking them after a hiatus of 1 to 3 years to let their bones recover.

CHAPTER 4

THE BACK PAIN SOLUTION

Prevention *to the rescue: The simplest, most-effective all-natural cures are something we all have the power to do, starting now.*

The spine is a thing of beauty: a sleek stack of 24 vertebrae, cushioned by 23 disks, neatly arranged into an elegant structure that's able to bend, twist, and shimmy at a whim. In a marvelous feat of biological engineering, it gives us both strength and flexibility. Yet back pain is rampant. Roughly 80 percent of Americans will experience it at some point, according to the National Institutes of Health. Why should this be? And what can we do about it?

PERFECT YOUR POSTURE

Esther Gokhale has a theory. A licensed acupuncturist, she says poor posture is a key culprit—one often overlooked by doctors. In her view, we slump most of the time. We sink into soft, cushy chairs that encourage us to round our backs rather than sit up straight. When not slouching, we're overarching or otherwise kinking our spines. Women lug purses the size of small suitcases and wear back-distorting high heels; men sit on thick wallets that nudge hips and lower backs out of alignment.

In workshops at the Gokhale Method Institute and across the country, she has helped thousands of sufferers by teaching them the proper ways to sit, stand, walk, and bend. Her approach is being heralded by some in the medical community as a promising new way to help prevent and treat chronic back pain without drugs, injections, or surgery.

Gokhale embarked on her quest for personal reasons. Pregnant with her first child in 1986, she suffered a herniated disk in her lower back that caused sciatic pain so intense that she couldn't sleep. She later had corrective surgery, but the pain returned within a year. Doctors recommended a second surgery and advised her not to have any more children.

Instead, Gokhale set out to create a remedy that would work better. She observed that back pain is much less common in nonindustrialized societies. Though it's hard to find precise statistics for countries where routine medical care isn't available, estimates for back pain in these societies are as low as 5 percent. At first, Gokhale thought that the reasons might involve trimmer figures and a more active lifestyle. Then she started noticing the people's beautiful posture.

LAUGH YOUR PAIN AWAY

The next time you throw out your back or do too many crunches, hit a comedy club or watch *Everybody Loves Raymond* reruns. Scientists at the University of Oxford in England found that a good laugh significantly raises pain tolerance by flooding the brain with endorphins, which are natural opioids that are produced in the central nervous system and can dull your pain as effectively as a pill.

BALMY DAYS AHEAD

Sore, achy muscles? Try a pain-relieving rub. These balms affect nerves in the skin, interfering with their ability to transmit pain to your brain. Caution: Don't combine hot packs with muscle rubs; it can irritate skin.

ICY HOT MAXIMUM STRENGTH MEDICATED PAIN RELIEF SPRAY ($8; drugstores): Has ingredients that start working on contact—no massaging required.

BADGER SORE MUSCLE RUB ($10; badgerbalm.com): Is USDA–certified organic and harnesses the natural power of cayenne pepper and ginger to bring you relief.

OLE HENRIKSEN MUSCLE COMFORT LOTION ($28; olehenriksen.com): Seaweed extract moisturizes, while peppermint oil cools and increases circulation.

BENGAY ZERO DEGREES ($14; drugstores): Goes on cold and has a scent that dissipates quickly.

In visits to a dozen countries, including India, Ecuador, and Thailand, Gokhale meticulously documented the way that the people carry themselves— erect, with an almost regal bearing, whether toiling in the fields, doing laundry by hand, or carrying heavy loads on their heads. Americans, on the other hand, scrunch. And we pay the price for our slovenly stance, Gokhale says, in back pain and also in sciatica, stiff necks, and paresthesia, or tingling in the arms and legs.

Gokhale traces the roots of our posture problem to an unlikely source: the devastation of World War I. To many at the time, the war represented the collapse of the old, aristocratic order, as the Austro-Hungarian, Ottoman, and Russian Empires crumbled. Afterward, styles of clothing and architecture became less stuffy and pretentious. Furniture followed suit, no longer encouraging the erect bearing of our upper-crust forebears but, rather, sultry flapper poses with rounded backs. Today we exacerbate the problem with all our modern gizmos, which have us staring down into screens on our laps rather than sitting up straight.

As evidence, Gokhale has amassed a library of photos showing how our great-grandparents 100 or more years ago maintained good posture, whether they were playing the banjo, sewing, or reading books to their children. She has photographed ancient Greek statues with much better alignment than we have today. She has even unearthed a pre–World War I anatomy book that shows the back much straighter than most modern depictions. While the basic S-shape of the spine is evident—rounded at the shoulders, arched in the lower back—the curves are less accentuated.

When it comes to spinal curvature, less is more, Gokhale says. Between those 24 vertebrae are disks shaped like hockey pucks. If the spine is erect, the disks maintain that pucklike form. But when you sway your back or hunch over your work, the tilted vertebrae squish the disks between them into wedge shapes.

Most of us tolerate this spinal abuse for decades. But after years of wear and tear, our backs can end up with herniated disks that bulge, compressing nerves in the spinal cord and leading to pain.

Bad posture can also put unnecessary stress on muscles and tendons, leading to stiffness and muscle strains.

FIGHT BACK PAIN IN YOUR SLEEP

You spend a third of your life in bed. But if you're not careful, you can twist yourself into contortions that irritate muscles or nerves.

THE FIX: A technique that acupuncturist Esther Gokhale calls "stretchlying" can help relieve pressure on nerves and disks. Here's how to do it. Lie on your back with a pillow under your knees. Prop yourself up on your elbows, and place your hands on your hips. As you slowly roll back down, one vertebra at a time, keep pushing your shoulders away from your hips to help lengthen your spine. Even if you spend just 15 minutes in this position, Gokhale says, "you're resetting the resting length of the muscles, and the nerves are decompressed."

"To quickly release tension in your upper back, do what I call the jellyfish stretch: Shake your arms like jelly to relax your muscles."

—Wayne Westcott, PhD, a strength-training consultant

POSTURE PERFECT

To improve your posture, focus on three main areas of your life: sitting, standing, and bending. Let's talk about each in turn.

Improving your posture can help prevent and relieve back pain, and Gokhale isn't the only one who thinks so.

"A lot of the gimmicks people spend money on—special chairs, every type of brace—don't really work," says Alexander Vaccaro, MD, PhD, a spine surgeon at the Rothman Institute in Philadelphia. "Good posture, with proper alignment, does."

Two doctors are now conducting pilot studies on Gokhale's techniques—one to see how they stack up against standard therapies and the other to measure changes in pain and flexibility.

Whatever the trials conclude, Gokhale's own back pain is a distant memory. Since that day 26 years ago when the doctor advised her not to have any more babies, she has borne two more children, with no back pain.

"Not even a twinge," she says.

Sit for success.

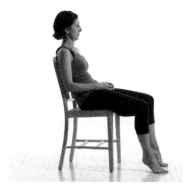

WRONG: Don't tuck your tailbone under, rounding your back. This can lead to lower-back pain. Similarly, hunching over your work or meals rather than leaning forward with a straight back places stress on neck and shoulder muscles, leading to stiffness.

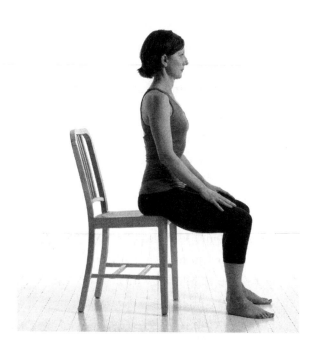

RIGHT. Straighten up, acupuncturist Esther Gokhale says. To flatten your mid-back, push gently on the bottom of your ribs. To align your shoulders, roll them up and back. And pull a tuft of hair gently back and up to straighten your neck. For extra length and support, tighten your core muscles.

Take a stand.

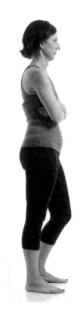

WRONG: There are so many ways to err, from sinking into one hip and rounding the upper back to the typical stance of someone told to stand straight: thrusting out the chest and swaying the lower back.

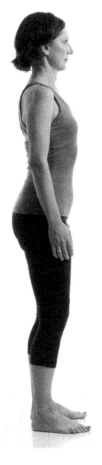

RIGHT: Flatten your spine as you would for sitting, says Gokhale. Make sure your weight is evenly distributed on both of your legs. Keep your knees soft to avoid sway in your lower back, and put your weight in your heels.

Bend better.

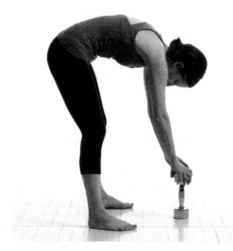

WRONG: When we stoop to make the bed or pick up toys and laundry, most of us crunch at the waist and round the lower and mid-back, compressing disks. Doing this repeatedly can lead to inflammation in the spine and cause impingement on nerves.

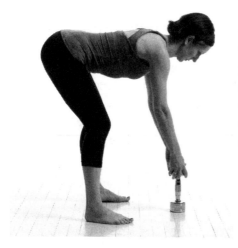

RIGHT: Keep your back flat, Gokhale says. The only way to do this is by tilting your hips forward. To get the feel of it, place your hands on your hip bones, with your fingers in front and your thumbs behind. Push down with your fingers, and let your body follow. Pick up only light objects this way.

MOVE MORE

Other research shows that moving more can be the best medicine for back pain. Here are two moves to send pain packing.

Stretching

What's the proof? A recent study found that stretching is just as effective as yoga at reducing back pain.

Why it works: Stretching of any kind, whether static (you hold the pose) or dynamic (you move through a complete range of motion), can help improve flexibility and decrease back-pain risk and symptoms.

Try this move: Half lunge, which stretches your hips and calves.

Stand with your feet staggered, your left leg in front. Bend your front knee about 90 degrees and lower your back knee a few inches from the floor. Press your right hip forward, feeling a stretch along the front of your hip. Hold for 20 to 30 seconds. Switch sides.

Yoga

What's the proof? Two recently published studies found that people who practiced yoga had less pain and more mobility than those who simply followed a self-care book on back-pain relief.

Why it works: Yoga combines stretching with strength and balance poses, which help shore up weak muscles and release tight ones. It's also a stress reliever; tension can lead to a tight back.

Try this move: Child's pose, which stretches your back and improves overall relaxation.

Sit on your heels, with your knees hip-distance apart. Exhale and lower your torso between your thighs. Reach your arms forward. Hold for about 30 to 60 seconds.

CHAPTER 5

24 WAYS TO BOOST YOUR IMMUNITY

From the latest research to time-honored remedies, here are the very best feel-good strategies for your healthiest year ever.

Here's a surprise: You might spend more time each year nursing a sore throat, fever, and runny nose than you do on vacation. Add it up: Adults get about three colds a year on average, each lasting a week or two. On top of that, 5 to 20 percent of us will also get the flu, which can linger even longer. That's a month—or more!

This year, take back that time—and your health. These tested tips for fighting colds and flu can help you stay well all year.

Meditate. Your mind can cut your chances of catching a cold by 40 to 50 percent, according to a 2012 University of Wisconsin, Madison study. Fifty-one people who used mindfulness techniques logged 13 fewer illnesses and 51 fewer sick days than a control group during one cold and flu season, probably because meditation reduces the physical effects of stress that can weaken the immune system.

Try probiotics. "We recommend taking probiotics—foods or supplements containing bacteria that are good for your health—that include Lactobacillus, because it can reduce the risk of both respiratory and gastrointestinal infections," recommends Mike Gleeson, PhD, professor of exercise biochemistry at Loughborough University in England. And people taking probiotics were 42 percent less likely to get a cold than those on a placebo, according to a 2011 meta-analysis of 10 studies.

Eat more garlic. "Allicin, a substance in crushed garlic, helps fight viruses," says Richard Nahas, MD, assistant professor of family medicine at the University of Ottawa. In a British study, volunteers who took a daily 180 milligrams allicin supplement caught 63 percent fewer colds over 12 weeks than those taking a placebo. Garlic cloves contain less allicin (5 to 9 milligrams), but even two raw cloves a day might help, says Randy Horwitz, MD, PhD, medical director of the Arizona Center for Integrative Medicine in Tucson.

Practice qigong. This Chinese mind-body exercise combines breath control and slow movements to reduce stress and improve focus, but it might also help combat colds. Twenty-seven varsity swimmers in a University of Virginia study learned qigong, and during their 7-week training season, those who practiced it at least once a week got 70 percent fewer respiratory infections than swimmers who used it less.

Exercise. People who exercise 5 or more days a week spend 43 percent fewer days with upper-respiratory infections, according to an Appalachian State University study.

You don't have to pump iron or train for a marathon to boost your immunity. Another study found that a regular 30-minute walk could slash your risk of catching a cold by 43 percent and make symptoms less severe, according to the *British Journal of Sports Medicine.* How? By increasing the circulation of cold-killing cells, says study author David Nieman, DrPH.

"I make sure I exercise to stay healthy," says Dr. Nieman. "Aim for 30 to 60 minutes daily. It boosts blood flow so that the immune cells circulate throughout the body."

Get vaccinated. "For flu protection, nothing is as directly effective as vaccination," says *Prevention* advisory board member David L. Katz, MD, MPH. If the post-shot muscle pain makes you injection-shy (and you're between ages 18 and 64), visit fluzone. com to find a location using intradermal shots, which are injected into skin and use much smaller needles.

Just 6 tablespoons of sugar can reduce your body's ability to fight off viruses.

Wash (and dry!) your hands often. Cleaning your hands frequently—especially after touching anyone or anything that might be germy—is key to defending yourself against cold and flu viruses. But drying hands thoroughly is just as important, because germs cling to your skin more easily when it's wet. Be sure to replace damp towels with dry ones often.

Get enough sleep. Your immune system needs rest to keep you healthy. In one study done at Carnegie Mellon University, even if people said they felt well rested if they'd averaged fewer than 7 hours of sleep per night, they were almost three times as likely to get a cold as those who got 8 hours or more of sack time.

Add astragalus. In test-tube studies, the root astragalus (uh-STRAG-uh-lus) activates T-cells, the white blood cells that fight off viruses, and experts believe it can prevent colds in real life too.

"Astragalus seems to work very well, and your body doesn't develop a tolerance to it, so you can eat it daily," Dr. Horwitz says. Use the earthy root as a vegetable, chopping up a 3-inch piece and adding it to soup. Or try 250 milligrams in standardized capsules twice a day.

Use herbs and spices. The oregano in your spaghetti sauce and the mustard on your turkey sandwich can boost your immune system, says *Prevention* advisory board member Tieraona Low Dog, MD, the author of *National Geographic's Life Is Your Best Medicine*. She suggests that you flavor bean and poultry dishes with oregano and thyme, and add ¼ teaspoon of turmeric to 1 cup of plain yogurt for a spicy dip.

Cut back on sweets. After people in a study at Loma Linda University consumed 6 tablespoons of sugar (whether in orange juice, honey, or sugary drinks), their infection-fighting white blood cells lost the ability to fend off bacteria and

SHOULD YOU GET A FLU SHOT?

Each winter, up to one in five Americans will get the flu, with more than 200,000 people sick enough to be hospitalized. Yet most of us still don't get vaccinated, often because of misconceptions about the shot. Here are four of the most common myths, along with the facts you need to know.

Myth: Only the elderly and those at high risk need to be immunized.

Fact: Influenza can make anyone, including the healthiest among us, seriously ill, and even if you don't develop symptoms yourself, you can pass the virus on to others.

Myth: The flu shot itself can give you a case of the flu.

Fact: The virus used in the vaccine is grown in chicken eggs and killed off before it reaches your bloodstream. There's absolutely nothing in it capable of causing a case of the flu.

Myth: You need a doctor's appointment for a shot. Who has time?

Fact: Drugstores and health clinics across the country provide walk-in vaccinations, and more and more local health organizations are setting up drive-through flu shot clinics.

Myth: If I have a cold, I should postpone getting a flu shot.

Fact: As long as you're not suffering from a major illness or running a temperature higher than 101°F, the flu shot doesn't present a health risk for you, according to experts.

viruses. Your immune system stays depressed for several hours after you eat or drink sugar, so if you down a soda every few hours (3 servings could put you over the 6-tablespoon mark), your resistance will be lowered for much of the day.

Lose weight. If you're carrying extra pounds, the flu vaccine won't work as well, and if you do get a bug, you're likely to become sicker. After vaccination, antibodies against the flu increase normally in obese people but decline prematurely over the next few months, lowering protection.

"If you're obese, be really vigilant about hand washing and other preventive measures," says Peter Mancuso, PhD, associate professor of environmental health sciences at the University of Michigan. "And even a 5 to 10 percent weight loss can help prevent all types of diseases."

Drink enough water. If you come down with a virus, your doctor might tell you to drink plenty of fluids to reduce your symptoms. But Jamey Wallace, MD, medical director at Bastyr Center for Natural Health in Seattle, says staying hydrated might stave off infections.

"Your mucous membranes and the immune cells in their secretions defend against cold viruses, and they can't work as well if you're dehydrated," says Dr. Wallace. His advice: Divide your weight by three. That's how many ounces of fluid you need daily, plus a glass of water for each caffeinated or alcoholic drink.

Take care of your toothbrush. Viruses on one toothbrush can contaminate others it touches. Make sure your family's brushes are in a holder that keeps them apart, and let them dry thoroughly. (If you get a bug, you don't need to replace your brush: You already have antibodies against that virus.)

Pop a vitamin C. A gram a day of this old standby does help alleviate colds, Dr. Nahas found in a review of studies about integrative approaches to preventing colds. In adults, the result is a modest 8 percent reduction in symptoms. It doesn't sound like much, "but that can shorten your cold by 1 to 2 days," he says.

Socialize. Even though people spread cold and flu germs, the more social relationships you have—family, friends, clubs, churches, volunteer groups—the less likely you are to get sick. Having a wide range of friends and acquaintances can provide psychological benefits—such as greater optimism and less depression—that boost the immune system, and they can also influence you to maintain good health habits, such as not smoking.

Stop biting your nails and wiping or rubbing your eyes or nose. You can't always avoid getting germs on your hands, but you don't have to give them a lift into your respiratory system.

"When you touch your mouth, nose, or eyes, you put the viruses right where they want to go to cause mischief," Dr. Nieman says. Keeping your hands where they belong sounds easy, but it's a challenge, he adds: Adults touch their faces about 15 times every hour.

Eat mushrooms. Many kinds of mushrooms might help boost immunity, but medicinal fungi such as shiitake, reishi, and maitake might be particularly beneficial because they encourage immune cells to multiply.

Take what you trust. Believing that a remedy is effective might make it actually work. In a study of echinacea as a cold remedy, people were told they were taking the herb, and those who believed strongly in its effects had shorter, milder colds—regardless of whether their pills were echinacea or a placebo.

"If there's a remedy your family's used for generations, and you believe in it and have used it before, by all means add it to your regimen," Dr. Nahas says.

Make your own sanitizing spray. To clean surfaces, mix 8 ounces of purified

THREE COLD TREATMENTS THAT REALLY WORK

If despite all your healthy eating, exercising, hand washing, and good hygiene, you've caught a cold, instead of reaching for a multisymptom "cold remedy," consider a more targeted treatment that won't leave you groggy or overmedicated. The following three products can help you recover faster and keep your illness from morphing into something worse.

CUT YOUR COLD SHORT. **Cold-Eeze:** Zinc lozenges can reduce your sick days. Researchers believe that the zinc ions bind to the same receptors in your throat and chest as the cold virus, which helps keep the bug from spreading.

STOP SINUS INFECTIONS. **Ocean Saline Nasal Spray:** By keeping your nasal passages moist, saline can help stop mucus from congealing and causing congestion and prevent germs from turning your cold into a sinus infection.

BANISH BRONCHITIS. **Halo Oral Spray:** Trials have shown that this product's antiseptic ingredients can keep your throat free of opportunistic bacteria, such as those that cause bronchitis, for up to 6 hours.

water and 30 drops of essential oil (try lavender, rose-mary, thyme, tea tree, or sage) in a spray bottle. Take aim at doorknobs, phones, or anyplace viruses are likely to linger, Dr. Low Dog says.

Be cautious about carriers. More than 8 percent of people without symptoms during cold and flu season are harboring cold viruses, according to a recent study from McMaster University in Ontario, Canada. The takeaway: When you're around others, wash your hands often.

...and things they might have touched. Flu viruses can live up to 8 hours on surfaces, so it's wise to clean whatever you can that might have been handled within that time frame. And think beyond the usual suspects: New research points to workplace hot spots such as vending-machine buttons and the handles on break-room faucets, microwaves, and shared refrigerators. Use a disinfectant wipe or tissue if you have to touch potentially contaminated objects, and don't forget to wash your hands afterward.

Eat more fruit. "We looked at everything people ate, but the impressive benefit of fruit just jumped out of the data," says Dr. Nieman, who also studied the effects of diet on colds. People who ate three or more servings daily had 25 percent fewer days with respiratory symptoms during cold and flu season than those who ate one or fewer. The vitamin C content might provide part of the punch, but fruit also contains polyphenols, which have antiviral properties.

Go green. Add another item to the list of reasons to eat your greens: Cruciferous vegetables such as kale seem to enhance the function of immune cells in the skin and the gut, according to the journal *Cell*. This is particularly important because it's these cells—especially the ones in the skin—that form the body's first line of defense against germs that cause colds and flu.

Check out our How to Prevent Anything center for more natural home remedies at prevention.com/prevent.

Natural DIY sanitizing sprays clean surfaces safely, and they can be misted to freshen the air too.

CHAPTER 6

ASLEEP AT THE WHEEL

We've all grown groggy with a foot on the gas. But what most of us don't know: This can be one of the deadliest driving risks we take. Writer Margot Gilman shares her story in her own words.

For as long as I live, there are certain things I know will never happen. I will never be talked into bungee jumping, for instance. Nor will I ever acquire a taste for maraschino cherries or be convinced to eliminate yoga pants from my wardrobe. I will never give up carbs. Until recently, I also would have said that in my life, I would never, ever fall asleep at the wheel of my car while going 65 miles per hour with both of my kids in the backseat. Not in a million years. But I was wrong.

I learned just how wrong I was on the day in August 2011 that Hurricane Irene was due to make its second US landfall and hammer the Northeast. Residents of eastern Long Island had been advised to evacuate, so I was driving my girls, then ages 11 and 14, and myself from our beach house back home to

New York City, where presumably we would be safer. Except for the looming threat of the biggest storm to hit the area in 73 years, it started off as a garden-variety summer Saturday. I woke early but refreshed after 8 hours of sleep and went off to take my usual 45-minute exercise class. My friend Ann and her two girls were visiting us at the beach house, and after breakfast, we all did some back-to-school shopping. Then we helped my husband, Steve, carry in the outdoor furniture, packed our bags, and began our drive in our two separate cars. (Steve stayed behind to deal with the potential for fallen trees and a flooded basement.)

Fifteen minutes into our drive, our little caravan stopped for lunch. Hurricane, schmurricane: Stomachs were grumbling, and pizza called! Sated on slices and soda, we got back on the road at about 2 o'clock. The day was warm, in the low 80s, and a light rain had just started. I left the windows rolled up against the drizzle but judged it not hot enough to turn on the air conditioner. My daughters popped in their earbuds. The car was cozy and quiet except for the low drone of the radio, tuned to hurricane talk.

The Long Island Expressway is about as dreary a highway as you could ever have the misfortune to drive: hill-less, curve-less, and charmless, lined with office parks and usually traffic clogged. About an hour into the trip, I began to feel drowsy in the way that many drivers know. Ironically, most nights at home, I have to set the stage for sleep, plumping my pillow just so, arranging the blankets, and deciding on happy thoughts to drift off to so anxious ones don't pop into my head and keep me awake. This tiredness just washed right over me; I didn't have to help it along. In the past, when I felt drowsy while driving, I

LIFESAVING CHEWS AND BREWS

To stay alert during long missions, US soldiers used to eat freeze-dried coffee grounds. But in 1999, the Army began research to find a way to deliver caffeine more efficiently.

The resulting product, Stay Alert chewing gum, is now available over the Internet. One piece delivers 100 milligrams of caffeine—similar to 12 ounces of coffee. But whereas the caffeine in brewed java must be absorbed through the stomach lining, which takes 30 minutes, the stimulant in the gum is absorbed via the lining of the mouth. After just 5 minutes of chewing, 85 percent of the caffeine hits your bloodstream, and 99 percent is absorbed within 10 minutes. To order, go to stayalertgum.com.

No gum on hand? Then drink the most caffeinated beverage you can find. Here is the amount of caffeine in some of the more high-test options, per 12-ounce serving:

HOW MUCH KICK IS IN YOUR CUP?

Starbucks Bold Coffee	260 milligrams
Generic brewed coffee	142 milligrams
Red Bull	111 milligrams
Black tea	71 milligrams
Mountain Dew	54 milligrams

SLEEP SOUNDLY

Here are two new ways to sleep better—before you next big car trip. Is there a long drive in your future?

MOVE OVER, WARM MILK. Tart cherry juice is the new potion for sweet dreams. People slept 39 minutes more after drinking tart cherry juice, according to a study in the *European Journal of Nutrition*. Researchers believe that the juice's high quotient of melatonin helps regulate sleep. Participants drank a 1-ounce dose of a concentrate in the morning and a second one before going to bed.

SLEEP BETTER, NO SWEAT! The cutting-edge technology that keeps you cool at the gym has made its way into the bedroom: Pajamas, sheets, and even mattresses are now made from sweat-wicking fabrics used in workout wear.

"These items move moisture away from your body so you don't wake up feeling clammy," explains sleep specialist Michael Breus, PhD. Two to try: sleep shirts from Wildbleu ($61; wildbleu.com) and Sheex Performance Sheets ($200 for a poly/spandex queen set; sheex.com).

opened the windows, blasted music, even slapped myself in the face. On one or two occasions, I pulled over to take a brief nap. This time, it all happened so fast that I hadn't gotten around to any of that.

The next thing I knew, my daughters were screaming. My eyes flew open to the sight and sickening sensation of my SUV slamming into a white van in front of me. I knew immediately that I had fallen asleep and that my reflexes and decisions in the next seconds would mean the difference between life and death.

Ann was on the road just behind me, and she later told me how she watched, helpless and horrified, as the scene unfolded. As if fused to the white van's rear bumper, my car hurtled down the highway along with it, fishtailing off to one side, then the other. Within seconds, my car broke free from the van and headed off perpendicular to traffic, straight at the cement barricade that divides west-bound traffic from east. We were still moving fast, and the tires screeched as I frantically jerked the wheel to the right, left, right. Amazingly, no one hit us as we careened from lane to lane. (Ann said other drivers took evasive action.) Thankfully, my car didn't flip before I was able to regain control of it. I hadn't dared breathe for the past 30 seconds, and now I gulped air and tightened my grip on the wheel to steady my hands. The driver of the white van pulled over in the right-hand shoulder, and somehow I managed to summon the nerve to change lanes and get behind him.

When I got out of my car, I broke down. "I fell asleep! I can't believe I fell asleep!" I remember wailing. I was traumatized and mortified all at once. My daughters were scared and crying but unhurt, and the driver of the van (a great guy who, seeing how shaken I was, tried to comfort me with a hug) was fine too. I have never been so thankful as when I realized that my car, not his, sustained all the damage. Still, I had come within a hair of killing my kids, myself, and God knows how many other people. How could I have done this?

Was I a bad driver? A bad mother? I needed to understand what had happened to me that day, and I've since learned that my crime, as it were, was that I didn't recognize how powerful a force sleepiness is. It's so potent that none of my usual tricks (loud music, cold air) could have been trusted to work.

"When your brain is sleepy, it can be very insistent," says Thomas J. Balkin, PhD, director of the behavioral biology program at the Walter Reed Army Institute of Research and a leading expert on sleep and fatigue. "When you've reached the stage where you are fighting sleep, the effect of any attempt to rouse yourself can be very short-lived." Even a shot of adrenaline—for example, the kind you feel when you drift out of your lane onto the rumble strips, as the vibration and noise scare you awake—won't help you for long.

"Yes, that shock makes you feel suddenly optimally alert," Dr. Balkin says. "You think there is no way you could fall asleep now, but that alertness lasts only about 30 seconds."

You force yourself awake, and to make matters worse, you can't really assess how sleepy you are.

"Sleepiness affects the part of the brain responsible for both judgment and

"When you've reached the stage where you are fighting sleep, the effect of any attempt to rouse yourself can be very short-lived."

self-awareness," says Dr. Balkin. As awareness drifts away, we do not, obviously, realize this is happening. "If you're driving, you may know you feel tired, but you do not know that you are falling asleep," he says. "It's completely insidious."

You can also fall asleep very briefly and wake up without even being aware that you nodded off. These "micro-sleeps" might last for just a few seconds—enough time for something awful to happen if you're behind the wheel of a fast-moving 2-ton vehicle. Researchers at the University of Wisconsin–Madison found that microsleeps occur when certain brain cells go briefly offline in a tired but still-awake brain. In other words, you don't have to be fully asleep to behave as if you are.

The only thing to do when you first feel drowsy while driving is to pull over immediately. If there is another driver in the car, hand over the keys. If not, get yourself a cup of coffee or another highly caffeinated beverage. Drink it, then let yourself take a 15-minute nap. The order sounds counterintuitive, but it takes about 30 minutes for the caffeine to work its way through the digestive tract and into your bloodstream, at which point, it will rouse you from your slumber. Researchers at Loughborough University in England found that combining caffeine and a nap was better at increasing alertness than either alone. They also found that just "taking a break" that did not involve caffeine or napping—even if it included exercise—was completely ineffective.

Still, the question remains: Why did I get so sleepy in the first place, in the middle of the afternoon, after 8 hours of sleep? It turns out that the circumstances of my day created a kind of perfect storm. According to Dr. Balkin, how much sleep you get on a regular basis—not what you got the night before—is a better indicator of your ability to stay alert during activities such as boring, monotonous drives. The fact is, I average only 6 hours of sleep a night. Our brains have a "sleep bank," Dr. Balkin says. Every day, we make deposits into it and withdrawals from it, and although there is some variability between people, studies show that those of us who average only 6 hours are generally sleepier (as measured by reaction-time tests) all day long than those who average 7 to 8, even if they claim (as I would have) to feel totally rested. My 2 hours of extra sleep the night before certainly added to my account, but not nearly enough to compensate for my overall sleep debt.

Nor was I aware that the time of day, the warm temperature in the car, and the fact that I had just eaten lunch all added risk. While most drivers worry about night trips, the afternoon has a sleep sweet spot too, thanks to the circadian rhythm, the body clock that rules all of us. Generally speaking, we experience increasing alertness during the course of the day until evening, when arousal begins to dip in order to promote sleep. The only other time of day that our circadian rhythm dips is midday, usually around 2 or 3 o'clock. Not coincidentally, a 2010 study by the American Automobile Association Foundation for Traffic Safety found that as many drivers reported falling asleep at the wheel in the afternoon hours as who reported falling asleep late at night. Warmth tends to spur underlying sleepiness, Dr. Balkin adds, and feeling sleepy after a meal is a universal experience in adults, because of chemical and hormonal changes that happen during digestion.

I've told my story many times, and not once to someone who couldn't relate. Quite a few people admit to having had similar near-miss experiences. According to a National Sleep Foundation Sleep in America poll, 60 percent of adult drivers say they have driven a vehicle while feeling drowsy in the past year, and more than a third have fallen asleep at the wheel. The AAA study found that 7 percent of all serious crashes, and 16.5 percent of fatal ones, involved driver fatigue. Nevertheless, while most people are aware of the dangers of driving while intoxicated, drowsy driving still doesn't quite set off the same alarm bells.

Let my story be the siren in your head. The next time you feel sleepy at the wheel of your car, do what I should have done and pull over immediately. Whatever you do, don't think that you are mightier than your body's need to shut your eyes. That's what I thought, and though I learned my lesson the hard way, I know that only luck kept it from being a far-harder lesson still.

The Courage of Couric

Anti-cancer warrior. Groundbreaking journalist. Doting mom. Compulsive Tweeter. For her newest act, Katie Couric is hard at work on her talk show where she shares her hard-won wisdom on how to be your own best health advocate.

"When it comes to cancer, people appreciate the opportunity to share with me, as someone who understands," Katie Couric says.

"I don't mean to sound morbid, but I'm hoping that 'cancer advocate' will be the first line of my obituary.

It's definitely what I'm proudest of. I think journalism serves people—I do. But on the other hand, the idea that I've actually saved a few lives along the way through advocacy is incredibly gratifying to me."

Not everybody can make such a claim, but Couric can. That's what having the nerve to cheerfully undergo the first on-air colonoscopy will do for you. After her *Today* show exam in March 2000, there was a 20 percent rise in colon cancer screenings nationwide, dubbed the "Couric Effect" by the *Archives of Internal Medicine* in 2003. "Whatever it takes," Couric says drily.

The reason for her very public push about colon cancer was once an extremely private one. As is now well known, her husband, Jay Monahan, died in late January 1998 at age 42, a casualty of colon cancer that went undetected until it had reached stage IV. He was among the unlucky 20 percent whose colorectal cancers are first discovered only once they have metastasized to distant organs. Their daughters, Elinor and Caroline (Carrie), were 6 and 2.

"Nothing fuels an education like fear and desperation," Couric says. During Monahan's illness, she says, "I would check every day, do a search, thinking something's going to come on the market." But time was not on their side.

By 2000, Couric had cofounded the National Colorectal Cancer Research Alliance, an arm of the Entertainment Industry Foundation, which has recruited the likes of Diane Keaton, Vanessa Williams, and Heidi Klum. Couric also cofounded the Jay Monahan Center for Gastrointestinal Health in 2004. And every March—National Colon Cancer Awareness Month since 2000—she has geared up to lobby, lecture, and sweetly hector us: Get screened. It's a no-brainer.

"I think people feel a real intimacy with me, which is nice."

Couric will be able to further spread the word with the help of her daytime talk show—called simply *Katie*. Her show features many segments on wellness and health, though she comments, "I'm not Dr. Oz." What she is, however, is a thoughtful, authentic voice when it comes to talking with real women about real life—a skill well honed in her 15 years as a cohost of *Today* and groundbreaking tenure as the first female solo host of an evening newscast, on CBS.

"I think people feel an intimacy with me, which is nice," Couric says. "When it comes to cancer, they appreciate the opportunity to share with someone who understands what they've experienced."

Prevention: You're a cofounder of Stand Up to Cancer, which is a nonprofit organization founded in 2008, whose goal is to bring together the best and the brightest to "encourage collaboration instead of competition." What led you to do so?

Couric: There's no reason to be greedy and just focus on colon cancer. I wanted to expand my efforts and raise money for cancers that were rarer and have a new approach that would yield results for a lot of different cancers. One of the most exciting things in research now is that it's not so organ specific. Something that might be quite effective for melanoma might also have results in, say, childhood brain tumors. They're examining pathways, the way cancer behaves, the way cells divide. In terms of worldwide deaths, cancer is expected to overtake heart disease and malaria. It's a real scourge. So we have to keep a foot on the gas pedal.

Prevention: And you especially liked the collaborative approach?

Couric: The world of cancer advocacy and research can sometimes be politicized. Part of it is human nature. People are competing to come up with the best treatment or drug. But it frustrated me that institutions are at times insulated from what other scientists are doing. It seems to me that a more-coordinated, collaborative paradigm would be helpful to everyone.

Initially, when Stand Up to Cancer wanted doctors from various institutions to work together, they were a little nervous about it. It was such an anomaly for them in terms of the business of cancer and the research that had heretofore been conducted. But after they got used to the idea, they were so excited. I think it reenergized them in a way they hadn't been in a long time.

Prevention: You have said that when someone you love is sick, it's important to not give up hope. Was that your experience with Jay?

Couric: I never acknowledged that I had given up hope. Sometimes I wish I had spoken with him about what we knew was inevitable. I really never had an opportunity to say good-bye to Jay, because I thought that accepting the fact that he was going to die—whether it was too painful or... I don't know. I wish I had been more honest. I was trying to protect him. Maybe I was trying to protect me. But for whatever reason, we never really acknowledged what we both knew to be true: that he was going to die. It was left unspoken, and as a result, a lot of things weren't said that I wish had been.

Prevention: This must make you very diligent about your own health, when it comes to your diet regimen.

Couric: I've always been a pretty healthy eater. I like to eat cereal that's high in fiber. I also try to take a multivitamin with folic acid, though I can't say that I remember to do it every single day [laughs]. My 18-year-old daughter, Carrie, is a vegetarian, and my diet has improved because of it. I eat a lot of black beans, a fair amount of fish, plus spinach and broccoli. I worry about my girls and try to make sure that they eat healthy too.

Prevention: What's your exercise routine?

Couric: I do Spinning and Pilates in the morning, between 8:30 and 10, maybe 4 or 5 times a week. I used to play tennis once a week, but I kept missing my class.

I want to get more into yoga this year. I think it's important for someone my age to stay flexible. And it's a great stress reducer. I've tried hot yoga, but it's pretty tough for me. I usually feel like I'm going to pass out.

Prevention: Speaking of your girls, Ellie and Carrie, what are you most pleased about as their mother?

Couric: I'm really proud of my daughters, and I know they're ambitious and want to make their mark on the world. They have a lot of confidence and poise, but I think what I'm proudest of is that they have really good manners. Parents don't realize that children observe how their parents treat other people and then behave accordingly. It really bothers my daughters if their friends are rude to waiters or cab drivers. I think it's because I've always made an effort to treat everyone respectfully, and my girls are a

> *"I want to get more into yoga this year. It's important to stay flexible."*

reflection of that. I'm especially proud when they meet people. They shake their hands, look them in the eye, and say, "Hi, I'm Carrie Monahan; so nice to meet you." It's so important.

Prevention: What lessons have you tried to teach the girls?

Couric: I try to set a good example in terms of dealing with failure or setbacks. I think one of the problems is a lot of parents—myself included—don't allow their kids to fail. Overparenting does a disservice, because we're not allowing kids to develop coping skills when they don't get perfect grades or win school elections. It's something that I think about.

Prevention: Do you think the girls are going to go into media, like you?

Couric: Ellie is figuring it out right now. She loves to write, and she's a very people-oriented person. She also teaches sex education and nutrition to kids in public school in New Haven. It's part of a Yale program. She might go to law school; her dad was a lawyer.

Carrie is pretty remarkable and incredibly smart as well. I don't know what she wants to do. She's only 18, so she has time. You want to guide them, but you don't want to push them in a particular direction, because you want them to have the opportunity to discover for themselves what they feel passionate about.

Prevention: Do they tweet as much as you do?

Couric: No, they don't. In fact, they get mortified when I do it. I think it's hard for them sometimes to have a mother who is a public figure and that people sometimes say not very complimentary things about. Carrie follows me, and I think Ellie does too—a lot of their friends follow me, so it's sort of fun. But they're not super into tweeting. They do enjoy Facebook, that's for sure.

> *"I try to set a good example in terms of dealing with failure or setbacks."*

Prevention: What do you think about the future of young women in America today? What sort of options do they have in society and politics?

Couric: It's a mixed bag. In some ways, I think women have more opportunity than ever before. In other ways, culturally, I feel like they're objectified as much as they ever were. In many places, sexism is still a much more accepted prejudice. I was watching an episode of *Mad Men* with Ellie, and Peggy was facing all these struggles as a copywriter. She was being iced out of a lot of meetings, and I thought, Well, gosh, that wouldn't happen today. But there are still subtle forms of sexism that exist that we have to be mindful of. We need to keep striving, because the more women who are in leadership positions, the more of a trickle-down effect is created. We've made tremendous progress, but there are miles to go before we sleep, as Robert Frost would say.

Prevention: You turned 57 in January, which makes you a Capricorn. Are you typical of the sign?

Couric: If they're hardworking, then I am. I know that my former executive producer, Rick Kaplan, told me that I still work like I don't have two nickels to rub together, which I took as a compliment!

Prevention: How is *Katie*, your talk show, shaping up?

Couric: We've got a notebook chockablock with ideas, and ABC has been wonderful. They seem to like the kind of work I do. One of the things I'm most excited about is being able to help people navigate or understand medical information or certain illnesses better through the show. If I can accomplish that, it'd be great. I've gone through a lot of medical situations, through Jay and my sister [Emily, who died in 2001 from pancreatic cancer], and my dad had Parkinson's. So I'm sort of the family advocate. I try to learn all I can to be helpful to my family members. I'm also very interested in health and wellness.

Prevention: Are you optimistic about finding love again?

Couric: Of course! I am a person who really enjoys having a partner. I'm pretty much a glass-half-full kind of person. That hasn't changed. (Editor's note: Couric got engaged in fall 2013.)

"I'm pretty much a glass-half-full kind of person. That hasn't changed."

Part 2

WEIGHT-LOSS
WISDOM

CHAPTER 7

SEVEN REASONS YOUR DIET'S NOT WORKING

Can't drop those extra pounds? The following surprising explanations can help you reach your goals.

You've spent the past 7 days putting in your best effort to lose a pound or two. But your weekly check-in with the scale reveals (again) that you can't get your weight-loss mojo in motion. The good news is that the problem probably isn't your willpower. You might be making common mistakes that even inveterate dieters fall prey to. Here are seven surprising reasons why your weight-loss plan isn't working. Get the facts and get back on track.

YOU AREN'T EATING ENOUGH

You might need to bump up your calorie intake to stoke your metabolism. When you dip below about 1,200 calories per day, you aren't eating enough to get all your nutrients, plus your body slows its rate of metabolism in order to hold on to precious calories, says Christine Gerbstadt, MD, RD, author of *The Doctor's Detox Diet*.

Also, if you skip meals to lose weight, your body could lose its ability to feel full. Blame evolution, which has designed our bodies to resist famine and not the buffet table. For example, if you skip breakfast, the body assumes that food is scarce. You need a morning meal to let your body know it's okay to burn calories.

"Within 1 hour of waking, you should consume a 350- to 500-calorie breakfast, with 10 to 15 grams of protein and fiber to stoke the metabolic fire," says Dr. Gerbstadt.

YOU REWARD YOURSELF WITH FOOD AFTER EXERCISE

Burning 300 calories during a workout is cause for celebration. But rewarding yourself with a high-calorie treat doesn't add up to weight loss. You're likely to overestimate how much the workout burned off and underestimate how much you ate.

"Even if you're just working out for well-being, you still have to keep calories in check," says Heidi Skolnik, author of *Nutrient Timing for Peak Performance*.

YOU SLURP DIET DRINKS

Research suggests that diet drinks might backfire: The taste of something sweet without the calories can cause your body to hold on to calories as fat. In a 2011 study, diet-soda drinkers had a 178 percent greater increase in waist circumference over 10 years, compared with non-diet-soda drinkers.

"Artificial sweeteners can actually raise your insulin levels and lower your blood sugar, which may stimulate hunger and move existing calories into storage in your fat cells," says Sharon P. Fowler, MPH, one of the study's coauthors. Plus, fake sweeteners might not quell a craving like real sugar can, because sugar triggers a longer dopamine release. So even after downing two Diet Cokes, you might still want the candy bar.

YOUR FRIENDS ARE FAT

Your chances of being overweight or obese increase half a percent with every friend in your network who is obese, found a 2010 study from Harvard. That more than adds up: Your chance of obesity doubles for every four obese friends you have, say researchers. Even if a friend lives thousands of miles away, your chance of gaining weight still goes up, according to a 2007 *New England Journal of Medicine* study. That might be because your perception of being overweight changes; living larger seems acceptable because the heavy person is a friend. (Interestingly, having an obese neighbor that you don't know does not raise your risk.) Experts also think that a person's lifestyle and behaviors can subconsciously rub off on those in the individual's inner circle.

But you don't have to ditch overweight friends to lose weight. In fact, if you embark together on an exercise plan, you can increase your fun and calorie burn: Research from Oxford finds that exercising with friends as a team can actually make the agony of exertion less intense. The same hormones that are released during social bonding, endorphins, also help quell pain. And once a friend starts to lose weight, you have a greater chance of losing as well because the mechanism works both ways.

YOU'VE ELIMINATED WINE

New research from Brigham and Women's Hospital in Boston found that women who drank one to two glasses of wine daily gained less weight over 13 years, compared with those who did not drink alcohol—8 pounds versus 5.5 pounds, to be exact.

YOUR DIET ISN'T DIGITALLY ENHANCED

You might already know that writing down what you eat helps you automatically reduce your calorie intake, simply by making you aware of each bite. But did you know that using a digitized program or application with positive feedback can help you lose even more? A new study from the University of Pittsburgh finds that people who monitored their diet and exercise with a digital device that provided daily feedback lost more weight and stuck with their diet longer than those who used paper and pen. Not only that, but the high-tech group increased their fruit and veggie intake more than paper users.

You don't have to log in daily or even weekly to benefit: One study found that dieters who recorded meals online just once a month were three times more likely to keep off pounds over 2 years, compared with those who did so less frequently.

YOU'VE GONE NO-CARB OR FAT-FREE

Cutting back markedly on any one food group—say, carbs or fat—can leave you short on the nutrients you need to stay energized. One study found that dieters low in calcium and vitamin C had higher odds of putting on belly fat.

The trick is a varied diet that includes healthy fats and good carbs such as fruits. After all, the biggest reason low-carb diets backfire is that, for the vast majority of people, they aren't sustainable over the long haul. It's a rare soul who can pass up birthday cake and pasta dinners for a lifetime. And as with all diets, once you quit, you regain the weight you lost and (often) more. These fluctuations can make it an even bigger challenge to lose weight next time.

THE HEALTHY WAY TO INDULGE

You can swear up and down that you won't overdo it, but when dessert rolls around at a holiday or special dinner, passing up cheesecake or pumpkin pie for a piece of fruit might be a lot harder than you expected.

"Before the holidays begin, pick out one or two of your favorite foods to indulge in a couple times over the course of the season," says Keri Glassman, RD, the author of *The New You and Improved Diet*—say, pumpkin pie or eggnog. "Then, when offered something you don't love, like gingerbread cookies, you can say no without feeling deprived." It's a simple way to avoid gaining hard-to-lose holiday weight this year.

CHAPTER 8

YOUR BELLY— LOVED AT ANY AGE

Don't have a six-pack? Who cares! Stop beating up your belly and learn to nurture and care for your core with this supersimple plan.

Muffin top. Pooch. Spare tire. Whatever you call the extra flesh around your middle, it's probably not flattering. But it's time we started giving our bellies a little love. After all, they're our core, the place where the magic happens—where babies grow, where nutrients get absorbed, and where gut feelings guide our choices.

Besides, most women aren't genetically programmed for washboard abs, and that fantasy becomes less attainable as we head through our forties and fifties, says Pamela Peeke, MD, *Prevention* advisory board member and the author of *Fight Fat after 40*. Why? Unless you make an effort to maintain muscle, you lose about half a pound of it every year after 30—and after 50, the rate doubles. Because muscle burns 6 to 9 calories per pound every day, your metabolism can slow substantially. Plus, as levels of estrogen and progesterone drop in your forties, your body stops storing fat in your hips and butt and starts packing it on in your gut.

"Even fit women can gain a few pounds around their middles," says Dr. Peeke. "Unless you're an elite athlete, you're probably not going to have flat abs."

What you can have is a healthy belly. And there are good reasons to try. There are two types of belly fat: the squishy outside layer, and visceral fat, a deeper type that builds up around the internal organs. The former can make you feel self-conscious; the latter increases the risks of everything from type 2

SHOW YOUR BELLY SOME LOVE

Fact of life: As we age, our bodies change, especially our bellies. Sure, it's hard to love those love handles, but if you appreciate your midsection, lumps and all, you're more likely to adopt the healthy habits that can keep it tightened and toned, says Ann Kearney-Cooke, PhD, coauthor of *The Life You Want*. Here's how.

STOP COMPARING YOURSELF TO A FANTASY. Those bare-abbed goddesses in the glossies are often the result of the fanciest digital fixes. "We've become conditioned to want things that aren't natural," says Sarah Maria, a body image expert and the author of *Love Your Body, Love Your Life*. "Teach yourself to value a natural body. Discover the beauty that comes from being alive."

STOP BELLY BASHING. "If you think, ugh, my belly is gross, ask yourself: Would I ever say that to a good friend?" says Vivian Diller, PhD, the author of *Face It: What Women Really Feel As Their Looks Change*. Instead, think of the ways your abdomen works for you, from keeping your immune system functioning well to gestating babies. "Gratitude is a great antidote to unhappiness," says Dr. Diller.

PROJECT FORWARD. "Ten years from now, you may really appreciate the belly you have today," says Dr. Diller. "Why not just appreciate it now?"

diabetes and heart disease to cancer. So keep yourself healthy by giving your belly the TLC it deserves. Get started today using our three-step process:

1. Your fitness plan
2. Your nutrition plan
3. Your lifestyle plan

1. YOUR FITNESS PLAN

Try this simple two-pronged approach.

Get your heart rate up. For burning harmful belly fat, nothing beats sweaty, heart-pounding, calorie-burning cardio.

"You need to burn calories to lose belly fat, and the quickest way to burn calories is to increase the intensity of your workouts," says Cris Slentz, PhD, an exercise physiologist at Duke University.

A great way to do so: interval training, alternating high-intensity bursts of exercise with moderate-intensity ones.

"Intense means what feels hard for you, whether it's brisk walking or a full-tilt sprint," says Dr. Peeke. The goal: Try to get at least 5 days of cardio a week, alternating between a day of moderate exercise (aim for 30 to 45 minutes) and a day of interval training (aim for 20 to 30 minutes, alternating between 30 seconds at a fast pace and 1 to 3 minutes at a moderate pace).

Maintain (or gain!) muscle. While you might want to lose body fat, you probably need to gain muscle. One of the easiest ways to do that is by strength training.

"Lean body mass drives your metabolic rate," says *Prevention* advisory board member Wayne Westcott, PhD, director of fitness research at Quincy College in Quincy, Massachusetts. Without strength training, age-related muscle loss can cause you to burn far fewer calories every day (up to 240—the amount in a bag of M&M's) by the time you're 60. Muscle burns more calories than fat, plus trained muscle, which has pumped-up cells, incinerates about 50 percent more than untrained muscle, says Dr. Westcott.

In other words, a 120-pound woman, who typically has about 45 pounds of muscle, could burn 135 more calories per day if her muscles were fit and strong.

In a recent study, Dr. Slentz and his colleagues found that people who did resistance training in addition to their aerobics routine lost more belly fat than those who did aerobics only. So aim to fit in two or three strength-training sessions a week. Include upper- and lower-body moves—such as squats, lunges, overhead presses, and biceps curls—to ensure you're hitting all the major muscle groups.

Here's a sample week-at-a-glance.

Day 1: Cardio: 30 to 45 minutes at a moderate intensity

Day 2: Strength-training

Day 3: Cardio: 20 to 30 minutes of interval training

Day 4: Cardio: 30 to 45 minutes at a moderate intensity

Day 5: Cardio: 20 to 30 minutes of interval training

Day 6: Strength-training

Day 7: Cardio: 30 to 45 minutes at a moderate intensity

Note: Aim to hit all major muscle groups, doing two or three sets of 12 repetitions of each exercise.

2. YOUR NUTRITION PLAN

Try the following simple solutions for eating smart.

Fill your plate with protein. One of your best defenses against age-related muscle loss is to eat enough protein, which contains amino acids that help build muscle, says Christine Gerbstadt, MD, RD, a spokesperson for the Academy of Nutrition and Dietetics. In fact, two studies of midlife dieters found that women who ate more protein lost less muscle than dieters who didn't pay attention to protein intake.

Overall, try to get at least 30 percent of your calories from lean protein sources, such as egg whites, chicken, and fish.

Nix mindless eating. For battling belly fat, the single best diet strategy is losing weight overall, and the simplest method is cutting calories. When researchers from the Harvard School of Public Health compared four weight-loss diets for 6 months, they found that participants lost about 14 percent of their abdominal fat and 16 percent of the dangerous visceral fat, no matter what type of diet

While you shouldn't loathe your soft stomach, a big belly does increase your risk of diabetes. For every 2 to 4 pounds of fat that you carry in your belly, your risk of developing prediabetes or type 2 diabetes rises by about 8 percent, says Ian Neeland, MD, a cardiology fellow at the University of Texas Southwestern Medical Center and coauthor of a study published in the *Journal of the American Medical Association*.

Fat you carry elsewhere on your body doesn't pose the same diabetes risk that belly fat does.

"Abdominal fat is different from other body fat," says Dr. Neeland. That's because belly fat secretes excessive amounts of free fatty acids and adipokines, which are substances that might be toxic to muscle, the liver, and insulin-producing cells of the pancreas. "This can worsen insulin resistance and impair cholesterol metabolism, which leads to an increased risk of diabetes and heart disease," he says.

Keeping your waist circumference less than 35 inches (40 inches for a man) reduces your risk.

they were on, as long as they restricted calories.

To lose weight at a safe rate of about a pound a week, aim to reduce your daily intake by about 500 calories. Just don't drop below 1,200 calories a day, or you'll risk slowing your metabolism.

Crack down on carbs. Another way to speed belly-fat loss is to limit refined carbs, such as white bread, crackers, bagels, and pretzels. These foods cause a sharp spike in insulin, which is a hormone that prompts your body to store fat in the abdomen and elsewhere.

Go for the good fats. More and more research suggests that monounsaturated fatty acids (MUFAs) can help prevent fat from settling around your midsection. Some good sources of MUFAs include nuts, avocados, and olives—their oils too.

"Aim to get 25 to 35 percent of your calories from fat, with the majority of those coming from good fat," says Karen Ansel, MS, RD, a spokesperson for the Academy of Nutrition and Dietetics.

Get plenty of fiber. In 2012, researchers from Wake Forest Baptist Medical Center found that people who ate the most fiber had the smallest accumulations of visceral fat. For every 10-gram increase in soluble fiber, the rate of visceral fat accumulation decreased almost 4 percent.

"It's clear that macronutrients might play a role in where fat is stored, but at this point, it's not clear why," says Kristen Hairston, MD, assistant professor of internal medicine and the study's lead researcher. Aim for at least 25 grams of fiber a day from healthy sources, such as black beans, chickpeas, vegetables, fruit, oatmeal, whole wheat bread, and brown rice.

REAL WOMAN, REAL LIFE STORY

NINA WALCHIRK is a financial management expert in her sixties. In her own words...

MY BELLY IS centered.

I've realized that aging gracefully requires the ability to accept and embrace the changes that come along with another year. For me, that's meant being okay with my softer, rounder belly. Despite the flaws, I've learned to love it. After my mother passed a few years ago, I revamped my entire lifestyle and became a vegetarian. I decided to focus on happiness instead of sadness and fear. The result: a slim belly and happier outlook.

I LOVE MY BELLY BECAUSE it helps keep me healthy.

MY BELLY FEELS BEST WHEN I'm in a beautiful dress, doing something fun or silly with friends.

MY FAVORITE HEALTHY-BELLY MEAL IS a superfood-packed smoothie. I toss in things such as kale, spinach, cucumbers, and apples and blend with ice.

MY LOVE-YOUR-BELLY SECRET IS to stop using deflating language. No one is perfect.

Give your gut what it needs. "As women age, they tend to develop more belly troubles, like bloating and gas, because gastric motility usually decreases with age," says Dr. Peeke.

What can help: regular exercise, along with eating fiber and probiotics to help maintain a healthy balance of gastrointestinal bacteria, as well as drinking plenty of water to aid digestion and beat bloat. Try to eat a serving of yogurt with live cultures every day. Other foods with probiotics include cultured milks such as kefir and fermented products such as sauerkraut, miso, and tempeh.

3. YOUR LIFESTYLE PLAN

Stress less, enjoy more with these life-altering ideas.

Get your z's. When Dr. Hairston and her colleagues looked at more than 1,000 people ages 18 to 81, they found that those who slept fewer than 5 hours a night gained more visceral fat over 5 years than those who slept 7 or 8.

Additionally, a study at the New York Obesity Research Center found that sleep-restricted people might eat as much as 300 calories more the next day.

"When you're tired, you're more likely to reach for high-calorie foods," says Marie-Pierre St-Onge, PhD, lead researcher of the study.

Cut down on couch time. Sitting can be hazardous to your waistline. The more you do it, the worse it is, according to a 2010 Australian study of more than 4,700 people.

"The best advice for losing belly fat is to accumulate as much physical activity as you can every day," says Nathan Johnson, PhD, senior lecturer in exercise and sport science at the University of Sydney and a spokesperson for Exercise & Sport Science Australia.

Try some effective stay-active strategies. Walk to a colleague's desk instead of sending an e-mail; use a printer on a different floor; move the wastebasket by your desk out of arm's reach; or reduce your TV time and replace it with anything active, such as a walk, housecleaning, or gardening.

"For every total hour of sitting, you need 10 minutes of movement," says Dr. Peeke, "so after every 10 minutes of sitting, get up and stand or walk for at least 1 to 2 minutes."

Chill out. Chronic stress causes the body to churn out too much cortisol, which is a hormone that promotes the accumulation of belly fat, according to Dr. Peeke.

"This toxic stress also stimulates your appetite for sugary, fatty foods," she says. "You never hear anyone say, 'I'm so stressed out, I need a salad.'"

Instead of reaching for some chips, take a walk, phone a friend, or do a mini-meditation. Close your eyes and inhale, then exhale, several times.

"It short-circuits the stress reaction," says Rick Hanson, PhD, the author of *Buddha's Brain: The Practical Neuroscience of Happiness, Love & Wisdom.*

Experience joy. When researchers in the Netherlands studied more than 2,000 people, they found that those who were depressed were more likely to

REAL WOMAN, REAL LIFE STORY

JUDI GELMAN is an FBI special agent in her fifties.

MY BELLY IS health.

During a difficult time in my late thirties and forties, I used food to cope with my emotions and packed about 50 pounds onto my typically slender frame. I felt terrible about myself and hated that the extra weight hid my previously special-agent-worthy belly that I'd worked so hard to achieve. Luckily, I got back into a healthy routine when my stepdaughter started training for admittance to the US Naval Academy. For support and my own motivation, we started taking boot camp classes together. I trained alongside her, doing sprints, pushups, and lunges. I finally started to feel like my old self again and dropped the weight. Now I have better abs than I did in my twenties!

I LOVE MY BELLY BECAUSE it reminds me to take care of myself. The more fat you have in your belly, the harder your heart has to work.

MY BELLY FEELS BEST WHEN I'm working out. I feel strong, empowered, and beautiful.

MY FAVORITE HEALTHY-BELLY MEAL IS oatmeal with blueberries, flaxseed, pomegranate seeds, and strawberries.

MY LOVE-YOUR-BELLY SECRET IS to not spend your life in the gym just to get a six-pack. Love your body at any size.

REAL WOMAN, REAL LIFE STORY

ROBIN NEWMAN is the director of Global Egg Donors and in her late fifties.

MY BELLY IS energy.

Being active is like brushing my teeth; it's just another part of my daily routine. But you'll never find me at the gym. Nature is responsible for sculpting my core. Spending time outdoors is a form of spirituality for me because it's refreshing for my mind and body. But because of my job, I spend at least 8 hours a day hunched over a computer, which drains my energy and mood. So to keep moving, I started using a treadmill desk. Walking at a 1.5-mph pace still allows me to talk and type as I engage my core.

I LOVE MY BELLY BECAUSE it's my core. Everything from gardening and yoga to making love and sitting up straight depends on the strength of my abs.

MY BELLY FEELS BEST WHEN I'm outdoors, feeling the breeze against me as I'm kayaking on the water, or my hair blowing in the wind while I bike on the beach.

MY FAVORITE HEALTHY-BELLY MEAL IS homegrown. I like to use herbs and produce from my garden.

MY LOVE-YOUR-BELLY SECRET IS thinking of exercise as something joyful and happy. It makes me want to do it more often. Find a fun activity that serves as fitness in disguise.

have a significant increase in belly fat 5 years later. Here are two likely reasons a blue mood leads to more belly bulge. First, depression has been linked to an increase in cortisol. Second, the illness saps motivation, making it harder to maintain healthy exercise and eating habits.

We love the following effective stay-happy strategies: Get daily exercise, which works as well as antidepressants for mild to moderate depression, and take time to slow down and notice the positive, even if it's a simple joy.

"When something good happens, whether you finish a load of laundry or notice a beautiful sunset, savor the experience and let those feelings sink in for at least 20 seconds," suggests Dr. Hanson. "It strengthens the brain's neural circuits for happiness."

CHAPTER 9

MYTH BUSTERS!

Here's why you can cross "chewing gum makes you skinny" and five more diet myths off your dieting to-do list.

Myths. Old wive's tales. Our lives are full of them, and there are plenty of myths about losing weight and eating right. Here we bust some of the most prevalent.

CHEWING GUM MAKES YOU SKINNY

If you pop mint gum between meals to help keep your eating in check, that habit could be backfiring, reveals new research published in the journal *Eating Behaviors*.

How? Turns out the lingering taste of mint can reduce the palatability of healthy food, say researchers from the University of Buffalo. Just like how a swig of OJ tastes rather unpleasant after you brush your teeth, so too does eating produce after you chew mint gum.

To arrive at this conclusion, researchers had participants undergo one of two experiments: chewing either mint or fruit-flavored gum before completing a food reinforcement task—a computer game meant to gauge how hard people are willing to work for food such as grapes and potato chips—or chewing the same flavors before every meal for several weeks.

The results: Chewing gum, no matter the flavor, decreased feelings of hunger. However—and here's the key—chewing mint-flavored gum reduced a participant's liking and intake of healthy foods afterward.

In other words, chewing mint gum is a short-term fix, not a long-term solution. Sure, you might feel less hungry for a bit, but when you do eat, you'll be more likely to grab a candy bar over a carrot.

Mint gum's not the only dubious diet trick to watch for.

WHOLE WHEAT BREAD IS YOUR BEST OPTION

Compared with white bread, whole wheat bread is just less bad, explains Michelle Davenport, PhD, a nutrition consultant for the University of California's San Francisco Medical Center.

"Your average slice of whole wheat bread has a higher glycemic index score than eight ounces of Coke," she says.

The solution? Opt for brands made with whole wheat flour and ones that contain at least four grams of fiber. Avoid anything that doesn't list "flour" or "wheat flour" as the first ingredient.

CUTTING FAT INTAKE HELPS YOU LOSE WEIGHT

No way, says *Prevention* advisor Ashley Koff, RD. "Healthy fats are critical to the right kind of weight loss," she says. "I love hemp seeds, chia seeds, avocado, walnuts, and organic soy."

EGGS ARE BAD

Can eggs cause coronary heart disease—or diabetes, or are they even worse than smoking? Whatever science has suggested, it's not totally true, says Dr. Davenport.

"It's okay to have up to one egg per day, though there is no recommended intake for eggs right now," she says. The healthiest ways to prepare your morning mainstay include sticking with water-based cooking methods such as boiling, poaching, or steaming, suggests Dr. Davenport.

YOU CAN'T GO WRONG WITH LOW-FAT FOODS

Not true. "When foods are processed to reduce fat content, they tend to increase in sugar," says Dr. Davenport. "And sugar, as research now indicates, is the true killer."

DIET SODA IS THE BEST ZERO-CALORIE OPTION

Nope, says Koff, it's water. In fact, research suggests that the more diet soda a person drinks, the greater their risk of becoming overweight. Plus, artificial sweeteners might disrupt the body's natural ability to regulate calorie intake based on the sweetness of foods, finds an animal study from Purdue University.

So do your diet a favor and stick with water. Or choose unsweetened herbal teas or add your own herbs and spices to plain H2O, suggests Koff. (If that doesn't do it for you, consider the "15 Healthy Drink Options" below.)

BONUS! 15 HEALTHY DRINK OPTIONS

Once upon a time, the term "juice cleanse" wasn't part of our national lexicon. A "Red Bull" was something you'd expect to find on a farm, not on a store shelf.

But companies keep launching new drinks because Americans keep guzzling them. Beverage World estimates that per capita consumption of nonalcoholic beverages (not including water) was about 116 gallons in 2010.

Many drinks are nothing more than a blood sugar spike waiting to happen. But sometimes you need a little flavor or (gasp!) fizz that water can't provide. So what then?

"Keep it simple," says Keri Glassman, RD, the author of *The New You and Improved Diet*. "Stick to natural ingredients, and use a small piece of fruit—

about 60 calories—as a reference for how much is reasonable to consume at once."

Here are 15 drinks you'll feel good about gulping.

Sparkling Ayala's Herbal Water

$1.59–$1.99; herbalwater.com, grocery stores

Favorite flavors: Lemongrass Mint Vanilla, Cinnamon Orange Peel

Calories: Zero

Perks: You'll add a splash of class (but not calories) to your day with these sparkling waters, which feature flavor combos you've never heard before.

Alo Drink

$1.99; Whole Foods

Favorite flavor: Escape (aloe, pineapple, guava, and sea buckthorn berry juice)

Calories: 70 per serving

Perks: This juice contains sea buckthorn berry, which boasts omega-3s, -6s, -7s, and -9s. Together, these aid digestion, regulate inflammation, and maintain healthy skin and muscle, says Vandana Sheth, RD, a spokesperson for the Academy of Nutrition and Dietetics.

PitayaPlus Super Juice

$2.99; Whole Foods

Favorite flavor: Pitaya + Lemon + Coconut Water

Calories: 70 per bottle

Perks: The pitaya's flesh and peel are potent sources of antioxidants. One bottle of this juice delivers the antioxidant equivalent of about 100 large blueberries and 25 percent of your daily fiber. Bonus: This company sources pitaya from small, family-owned farms in Nicaragua and operates out of a solar-powered factory.

AhhMigo

$2.99; ahhmigo.com

Favorite flavor: Camu & Water

Calories: 20 per bottle

Perks: The star ingredient in this berry juice blend, camu camu berry, is a great natural source of vitamin C. One bottle contains 200 percent of your recommended daily intake. It's sweetened with a hint of maple sugar.

Mamma Chia

$3.49; grocery stores

Favorite flavors: Blackberry Hibiscus, Grapefruit Ginger

Calories: 120 per bottle

Perks: Thanks to chia seeds, each bottle contains 4 grams of complete protein and 25 percent of your recommended daily intake of fiber. These seeds develop a gelatinous texture when submerged in liquid, creating a smoothie-like consistency.

Celestial Seasonings Kombucha

$2.99; grocery stores

Favorite flavor: Original

Calories: 30 to 40 per serving

Perks: Kombucha is created by combining organic black tea, natural sugars, and SCOBY (symbiotic culture of bacteria and yeast). The SCOBY consumes the sugar, producing an effervescent drink containing probiotics, B vitamins, and acetic acid, which studies have shown can help stabilize blood glucose levels and boost satiety. Kombucha is raw and unpasteurized, so keep it refrigerated and consume within a few days of buying.

KeVita

$3.49; grocery stores

Favorite flavors: Mango Coconut, Pomegranate

Calories: 10 to 90 per bottle

Perks: These organic blends of fruit juices and seltzer are lightly sweetened with stevia and contain probiotics—4 billion colony-forming units at time of manufacture—to help maintain a healthy gut.

Tea of a Kind

$2.99; teaofakind.com

Favorite flavor: Peach Ginger Black Tea

Calories: 10 per serving

Perks: This tea's bottle cap contains a special pressurized chamber that self-mixes the tea when you twist the cap, which may help preserve antioxidants (plus, it's fun to open!). It's lightly sweetened with stevia and a bit of cane sugar.

The Republic of Tea Iced Tea

$5; republicoftea.com

Favorite flavors: Mango Ceylon, Blackberry Sage

Calories: Zero

Perks: This sophisticated black tea features natural, exotic fruit flavors and contains no added sweeteners. It's not too strong and provides just the right amount of caffeine for a slight energy boost.

Cheribundi

$2.49; cheribundi.com, grocery stores

Favorite flavor: Skinny Cherry

Calories: 90 per bottle

Perks: Eight to 12 ounces twice a day of tart cherry juice—a favorite among elite athletes—has been shown to boost muscle recovery after exercise and reduce inflammation, which means it might help with achy, arthritic joints. This juice is lightly sweetened with stevia and has the nutritional power of 40 cherries.

Zukay Kvass

$3.49–3.99; Whole Foods, Wegmans, natural food stores

Favorite flavor: Super Gold

Calories: 35 per serving

Perks: Kvass is a common Eastern European fermented drink. This sweet and spicy variety contains probiotic cultures, antioxidant-rich yellow veggies such as winter squash, and the spices turmeric and ginger, both of which have anti-inflammatory properties. Like kombucha, kvass is raw and unpasteurized.

Izze Esque

$1.39–$1.69; Whole Foods

Favorite flavor: Sparkling Black Raspberry

Calories: 50 per bottle

Perks: If you want juice without all the calories, opt for this one blended with sparkling water. It contains just 25 percent of the calories of an equal amount of juice.

Taste Nirvana's All Natural Real Coconut Water with Pulp

$1.08; tastenirvana.com, grocery stores

Calories: 75 per bottle

Perks: This coconut water has 600 milligrams of hydrating potassium (about 180 milligrams more than a medium banana), so it might be a better replenishing option than a sports drink after an intense workout, says Glassman.

Numi Organic Pu-erh Bottled Iced Tea

$1.99–$2.99; numitea.com, grocery stores

Favorite flavor: Earl Grey

Calories: 40 per bottle

Perks: Pu-erh is a variety of tea that's fermented and aged for a prolonged period, similar to wine, and contains high levels of antioxidants. Some consider it to have a richer, smoother taste than other teas. This bottled variety is lightly sweetened with sugar.

Hint Fizz

$1.79; drinkhint.com, grocery stores

Favorite flavors: Blackberry, Peach

Calories: Zero

Perks: For a bit of flavor but nothing sweet, this sparkling water is the perfect blend of bubbles and natural fruit flavors. It has all the hydrating benefits of water but is way more fun.

CHAPTER 10

THE TRUTH ABOUT SUGAR

Scientists say that eating too much of the sweet stuff might be destroying our health. But can a normal American family really learn to survive on less? Writer Heather Millar explains in her own words.

The morning I decide my family will finally start the low-sugar regimen I've been threatening them with, things are, to say the least, rocky. When I remind my husband, Pete, that for the next 2 weeks, he's off his usual breakfast of sugary cereal, he looks at me as if I've punched him in the gut. I point out that it's not just the cereal itself—Rice Chex on a good day, but often, Frosted Flakes—but the fact that he adds 2 tablespoons of sugar on top, plus 3 more in his coffee. Those extra spoonfuls total around 63 grams of sugar—about 16 big sugar cubes—before you even get to what's in his cereal, milk, and orange juice.

He looks at me skeptically. "You know why people like junk food?" he asks. "Because it tastes good."

When my daughter, Erin, wakes up, I tell her that we're starting the sugar

"We made dessert a
treat rather than an
everyday routine."

experiment. "Not today!" she cries. "Tomorrow!"

I insist. She says it's not fair. I ask gently if she realizes that she sounds like an addict. She starts to cry, and then throws a pillow at me.

I go to the kitchen and cut up some strawberries and bananas. I toast a piece of whole wheat bread, spread it with no-sugar peanut butter, and top it with more sliced strawberries. I put the food in front of her. She looks at me as if I'd just killed a litter of kittens.

"These are all things you like," I say. "Please eat. Or don't. But this is what's for breakfast." I can feel the waves of hostility following me as I walk out of the room.

So why have I decided to put my family through this torture? Here's the deal: Americans are eating a lot of sugar—on average, about 130 pounds a year. To put that in perspective: In boxing, that's the same weight as a junior lightweight—a whole person, with muscles.

That's far more than we used to eat, and much of it is from processed foods. In 1986, the last year the FDA formally studied the impact of "added" sugar (that's what manufacturers put in food, not what's naturally in, say, apples or carrots), Americans were eating 150 to 200 calories of added sugar a day. That's 50 grams, or a little more than what's in one can of Coke—and far less than what Pete's standard breakfast contains. Today, Americans consume an average of 450 calories a day as added sugar, approximately one-quarter of a 2,000-calorie diet.

The increase is partly because we're eating more plain old sugar (or sucrose, which is made up of half fructose, half glucose). But it's also due in large part to the invention of high-fructose corn syrup, a form of grain-derived syrup that's been chemically manipulated to change some of its glucose molecules into sweeter-tasting fructose molecules, until the final product is about 55 percent fructose. HFCS really took off in the late 1970s, and it was added to all kinds of foods because it increases shelf life, makes low-fat processed foods and baked goods taste better, and is cheaper than regular sugar. It's become a staple of most of our oversweetened diets.

THIS IS YOUR BODY ON FRUCTOSE

What's supposed to happen: When you need to eat, your stomach produces a hormone called ghrelin to signal your brain that you're hungry. As you start eating, your pancreas releases another hormone called insulin, which enables your body to store glucose (which you get from food) as fat. Finally, in response to the insulin, your fat cells send out a third hormone, leptin, which travels to your brain to tell it to decrease your appetite. When everything works, you're unlikely to overeat, and you can burn energy properly.

If you eat too much glucose, the subsequent insulin rise can make you put on weight. But, according to endocrinologist Robert Lustig, MD, large amounts of fructose are what really wreak havoc on your system. Although both glucose and fructose are types of sugar, fructose doesn't stimulate the pancreas to release insulin the way glucose does, and it doesn't cause ghrelin levels to drop or leptin levels to rise, so your body doesn't know when it's had enough. Without those internal controls, you're liable to gain weight.

Regularly consuming lots of fructose also causes your liver to accumulate fat, which makes it resistant to insulin. To compensate, your pancreas has to release more and more insulin, until finally this large, overworked gland burns out, sugar collects in your blood, and you have type 2 diabetes. What's more, the strain on your liver can lead to high blood pressure, lipid buildup, heart disease, and more abdominal ("bad") fat.

Finally, fructose might also reduce your enjoyment of food. Dopamine, which is a neurotransmitter, signals pleasure. New research shows that if you eat too much fructose, you tamp down your dopamine receptors so that it takes more and more fructose to feel pleasure. That's how sugar can easily become an addiction, which is exactly why it's so hard to give up.

"No way am I going to get my peeps to eat squash hash browns."

But while our sugar consumption has been skyrocketing, so have rates of obesity, diabetes, lipid problems, high blood pressure, and heart disease, collectively termed metabolic syndrome, and research is starting to show that that's not a coincidence. Robert Lustig, MD, a pediatric endocrinologist and researcher at the University of California, San Francisco—and one of my neighbors—has been studying the biochemical effects of sugar on our bodies for more than 16 years. His conclusion: Sugar is a toxin that's fueling a global obesity pandemic, and it's why we all, on average, weigh 25 pounds more today than people did 25 years ago.

"The dose determines the poison. A little sugar is okay; a lot is not," says Dr. Lustig. "What that means varies from person to person. Everyone has a different threshold, but the majority of us are way over that threshold."

He makes a pretty convincing case. It's not just the calories in the sugar that are making us fat. It's the fact that consuming megadoses of fructose interferes with our hormones, our digestive systems, our brains, and our bodies' natural ability to regulate appetite—so we just keep eating. (See "This Is Your Body on Fructose" on page 91.) While glucose, a simple form of sugar found in plants, is a fuel source that almost every cell in our body needs, fructose is found naturally only in small quantities and usually in fruits that contain fiber, which helps limit how much fructose the body absorbs and how quickly. Our bodies don't need fructose at all, but we're consuming huge quantities of the stuff. The

AN AMERICAN'S AVERAGE DAILY SUGAR INTAKE

One sugar cube equals **4 grams of sugar.** Here's how much we eat, on average.

1950s: **34 sugar cubes per day.** High-fructose corn syrup wasn't widely used in the United States until **1977.**

1980s: **39 sugar cubes; 6 teaspoons of HFCS per day.**

Today: **47 sugar cubes; 10 teaspoons of HFCS per day.**

result? Despite our best efforts, we're getting fatter and sicker than ever.

Convincing people to give up sugar is a tough fight, but Dr. Lustig is gaining an audience. His 90-minute 2009 YouTube video, *Sugar: The Bitter Truth*, has been viewed more than 3 million times. He expands on those ideas in his new UCSF/YouTube video series called *The Skinny on Obesity*. He's written a new book, *Fat Chance: Beating the Odds against Sugar, Processed Food, Obesity, and Disease*.

I really don't think my family eats that badly. Really. I like to cook and eat a mostly healthy diet and try to make sure my family does too. But I've never encountered a baguette, roll, plate of pasta, or glass of wine that didn't sing a siren song to me. As for my husband, when I was pregnant, Pete swore that he'd give up Coke, Oreos, and Frosted Flakes so our daughter wouldn't start out with a less-than-perfect dietary role model. That lasted about a month. Erin, now 12, eats a reasonably balanced diet but, since she first trick-or-treated at 18 months, she has devoted her life to the pursuit of sugar. She hoards it, whines for it, and sneaks it when she can. Thankfully, she doesn't like sugared soda, but she loves juices, which Dr. Lustig says are just as bad for you, because they contain so much concentrated fructose—and none of the fiber that can help counteract it.

So I know we're not perfect. And Dr. Lustig tells me that the vicious hormonal cycles caused by excessive sugar consumption affect more than half of the US population—those who are obese, but also many who are normal weight. And the more I think about how impossible it seems to reduce my family's sugar intake, the more important it seems to make it work. So that's why my suddenly sugar-deprived family now hates me: We're going to live by the following rules for the next 2 weeks.

- Try to limit daily "added sugar" to the equivalent of 200 calories.
- Make sure carbohydrate-heavy foods—bread, pasta—have at least 3 grams of fiber per 100 calories.
- Stay away from packaged, processed foods. (That's where all of the added sugar is.)
- Limit desserts, refined pasta, and white bread to once a week as treats.
- Give up all sugary soda and juice.

DAY 3

We're settling into a rhythm.

The drama has abated. On weekday mornings, Dr. Lustig's family eats whole grain toast with fruit or steel-cut oatmeal. These options won't hold my family for long, so I put a shout-out on Facebook, begging for low-sugar, low-refined-carb breakfast alternatives. Friends come out of the woodwork with ideas: whole grain muffins; breakfast burritos with whole wheat tortillas; egg dishes of every kind; polenta (cornmeal mush) with cheese. A high school pal suggests squash hash browns, noting that salty-crunchy things can help with sugar withdrawal, which, Dr. Lustig tells me, is a real thing, because fructose has an addictive effect on the body.

Some are good ideas, and most of them work out well, but there's no way I'm going to get my peeps to eat squash hash browns. You've got to be realistic, and the food has to be good. Otherwise, your family will not stick with the program.

DAY 4

It's a Saturday.

I spend the morning cooking low-sugar alternatives such as microwave applesauce. (Supereasy: Peel and cut up apples; add water, lemon juice, and a little sugar and cinnamon; zap 10 minutes; mash; cool.) As Dr. Lustig's wife advises, I cut the sugar in my muffin recipes by one-third. I use 25 percent whole wheat flour instead of all white to add fiber. No one even notices.

The downside to eating less sugar is that it takes more time than most of us spend now getting a meal together. One recent study found that 80 percent of the 600,000 food items sold in American supermarkets have added sugar, most of them convenience foods. (Ironically, while people think processed foods cost less, Adam Drewnowski, PhD, epidemiologist at the University of Washington, has found that that's not true.) In the past, I checked labels only for calories, and I'm shocked at where I find sugar: in salami, in flavorings, in frozen french fries, in every cracker in our

"I cut the sugar in my muffin recipes by one-third. No one notices."

OUR MORNING MEAL MAKEOVER

Breakfast doesn't have to be so sugar saturated. Here's how our family cut back.

Before: We ate sugary oatmeal and cereal, orange juice, bagels with jelly—our breakfasts were as sweet as dessert! On a typical day, our family's combined sugar count was the equivalent of 22 sugar cubes!

After: Steel-cut oatmeal with fruit and nuts, whole wheat toast with no-sugar peanut butter, plain yogurt with berries, and milk are just as satisfying—and healthier! Our family's combined sugar count was now the equivalent of 12 sugar cubes.

cupboard, and even in ramen noodles.

"Parents are always saying it takes longer and costs more to prepare meals from whole foods," Dr. Lustig says. "But it's your time or your health; your wallet or your health."

Okay, I'm willing to put in my time at the stove, but I do it the smart way. I plan ahead. When I make dinner, I also prepare ingredients for the next day, simmering whole grains, soaking beans, and roasting squash so I'll have a head start on the next meal.

DAY 6

The day begins with victories.

Pete says that he doesn't really miss the full-sugar Coke. He's knows it's bad for him, so he's going to give it up. I made a big batch of whole grain bran muffins, and he says they're a pretty good alternative to his usual sugary cereal. Erin announces that she really likes barley. I've been pouring water or milk for my daughter to drink at meals, and she doesn't complain.

HOW MUCH SUGAR IS IN THAT?

The sweet stuff—both natural and added—lurks everywhere.

See how sugar-savvy you are. You'll find added sugar in beverages, food and snacks.

- Chocolate milkshake, 10.6 ounces (small): 62 grams
- White chocolate candy, ½ cup: 50 grams
- Raisins, ½ cup: 43 grams
- Gummy worms, 10 worms: 43 grams
- Fruited yogurt, 8 ounces: 43 grams
- Milky Way candy bar: 36 grams
- Grape juice (unsweetened), 1 cup: 35 grams
- Cola or Sprite, 12-ounce can: 33 grams
- Piña colada, 4.5 ounces: 31.5 grams
- Orange juice (unsweetened), 1 cup: 20 grams
- Applesauce (sweetened), ½ cup: 19 grams
- Vanilla pudding, ½ cup: 19 grams
- Sweet-and-sour chicken frozen entree: 16 grams
- Blueberry muffin: 15.5 grams
- Granola, ½ cup: 13 grams
- Carrot juice (unsweetened), 1 cup: 9 grams
- Banana, ½ cup: 9 grams
- Fast-food double cheeseburger on bun: 9 grams
- Plain cake doughnut: 8 grams
- Spaghetti sauce, ½ cup: 7 grams
- Sugar cube: 4 grams
- Pasta, 2 ounces: 2 grams

DAY 9

I'm beginning to notice that I have more energy. My breakfast stays with me longer. I'm hardly snacking at all, because I'm not hungry between meals. I've stopped reaching for bread or pasta every time I sit down at the table. I still like all those things, but it's not killing me to eat them less.

DAY 10

I desperately need to go grocery shopping, but I don't have time. I give Erin canned chicken soup for her school lunch. It has 4 grams of sugar—that's a little less than one Oreo. We're out of whole wheat bread, so I put in a sourdough roll. I do pack iced herbal tea instead of juice, but this lunch is a failure, sugarwise. Note to self: Plan ahead better.

DAY 11

We have friends over for dinner and go completely off the reservation: potatoes au gratin, cheesy cracker hors d'oeuvres, and so on. The good news: One guest brings a Chocolate Oblivion Truffle Torte. She says it doesn't have much added sugar, and when I look up the recipe in *The Cake Bible*, I realize she's right: It's just chocolate, eggs, and butter. It has about 10 grams of sugar per serving—not bad for a dessert. I never would have imagined that it's healthier to eat chocolate straight!

Dr. Lustig recommends indulging in this sort of thing once a week at most, and, I have to admit, it feels like such a treat. "That's the way it was a generation ago," he tells me. "People didn't have dessert at every meal."

DAY 12

The grocery situation grows dire. I get a press release from the American Heart Association about heart-healthy, low-sugar dishes, and I try to make the Greek salad recipe that calls for grated raw zucchini. Don't do this with zucchini that's been in your fridge for 2 weeks. That attempt goes straight to the compost.

Another lesson learned: If you're going to really go low sugar, high fiber, you've got to replenish your produce every 4 to 5 days—or have lots of recipes for frozen veggies.

DAY 13

Finally, I get to the store. As I walk in, though, I see it with new eyes: Everything—everything—seems to be screaming, "Sugar, sugar, sugar!" Shelves of cakes, breads, and cookies in the front; aisle after aisle of convenience foods, ice cream, juice, soda, candy, cereal, snacks, and so on. The real food—fruits, veggies, meat, milk, eggs, whole grains—exists on the fringes of the average supermarket. I barely enter the center aisles.

DAY 14

We made it! Erin is perfectly happy with the whole wheat peanut butter toast and strawberries that began a tantrum at the beginning. I feel like we've done a

Q&A

Q: Is agave nectar healthier than table sugar?

A: No. Unlike blackstrap molasses, for example, it doesn't offer more antioxidants or minerals. Its main advantage is that it's 40 percent sweeter than sugar, so you should be able to use less, reducing calorie intake. It might be a good option for people with diabetes because it has a lower glycemic load than other sweeteners, meaning it will cause less-dramatic spikes in blood sugar.

But like any sweetener, "if used in large amounts, it's not healthy," says Andrew Weil, MD, director of the Arizona Center for Integrative Medicine.

The bottom line: If you like agave nectar, use it, but try to use less sweetener in general.

real diet reset: Our table will feature more grains and proteins and fewer cookies, crackers, and cakes than before.

So did we stick to our 200 calories a day from sugar? Honestly, I couldn't keep up with all of the math, so I'm not totally sure. Let's just say that my family ate drastically less sugar, especially at breakfast. We made dessert a treat rather than a daily routine. We ate more whole foods with more fiber. We probably had pasta and white bread more than once a week, but we didn't have nearly as much as we used to.

And maybe the biggest discovery of all: After the initial shock, it wasn't that difficult. It took a little more time, and the fresh fruit cost a little bit more than cookies, but we felt good. After about 10 days, we stopped thinking about sugar, and Pete even stopped making sugar jokes. Erin seemed calmer, less hyper.

On day 15, I buy Pete a small box of Frosted Flakes as a thank you. He doesn't realize what day it is and opts for a bran muffin instead. I don't say anything. Maybe an experiment can become a lifestyle.

CHAPTER 11

YOGA FOR WEIGHT LOSS AND INNER HAPPINESS

Lighter, happier, more joyful. Yes, you. Boost your bliss and flatten your belly with our yoga plan. You'll drop up to 13 pounds in 6 weeks!

If you'd like to slim your belly and brighten your mood, look no further: Our Yoga for Weight Loss and Inner Happiness Plan does both in less than 30 minutes a day. The secret to its success is a Power Yoga routine and Joy-Boosting Journaling assignments, created by certified yoga instructor and counselor Ashley Turner.

Why this mix? Yoga is a fantastic way to reduce stress, ease aches, and boost

YOUR YOGA FOR WEIGHT LOSS
AND INNER HAPPINESS PLAN

Aim to do five or six Happy and Healthy Power Yoga sessions (see page 103) each week. In addition, do 15 minutes of Joy-Boosting Journaling (see page 111) daily. Swap days according to your schedule.

ACTIVITY	DAY 1	DAY 2	DAY 3	DAY 4	DAY 5	DAY 6	DAY 7
HAPPY AND HEALTHY POWER YOGA	X	X		X		X	X
JOY-BOOSTING JOURNALING	X	X	X	X	X	X	X

your energy levels—all of which add up to a healthier, happier you—and it can brighten your mood. A Boston University School of Medicine study found that participants who practiced yoga for an hour three times a week for 3 months had higher levels of the mood-boosting brain chemical gamma-aminobutyric acid than participants who walked for the same amount of time. The journaling exercises, meanwhile, build self-confidence and self-acceptance, while helping you pinpoint your true dreams and desires. The result: You become a more authentic, happier version of yourself.

But don't take our word for it. Listen to some of the 22 women over 40 we enlisted to follow this program plus healthy eating guidelines from nutritional educator and chef Missy Costello. (Find her tips at prevention.com/yogamenu.) After 6 weeks, the women felt happier and more energetic and lost an average of 6 pounds—some more than twice that.

"The changes I have seen in my mood and energy levels since I began this adventure are surprising," says Wendy Carter, a mom and stylist. "I am more energized and much more positive. As far as my body goes, all I can say is 'Holy cow!' I cannot believe I am down 13 pounds and 11 inches. Most important, this program helped me realize that I really like me. I will take care of my body for the rest of my life."

Diane Schmiedeke lost 7 pounds, but results on the scale weren't her main motivator. "This process changed my focus from becoming skinny to becoming healthy," Schmiedeke says. "I now feel more confident and less stressed too." Ready to get started? Read on!

HAPPY AND HEALTHY POWER YOGA

How to do it: Roll out your yoga mat on a firm surface. Then do our Happy and Healthy Power Yoga sequence. (See page 104.) Complete as many repetitions of each pose as possible, and continue to add reps as you become stronger and more familiar with the sequence. Throughout each pose, deeply breathe in and out through your nose. After completing the sequence, lie on your back for at least 2 minutes with your feet spread slightly apart, arms by your sides, and eyes closed.

What you'll need: A basic yoga mat. Our testers used the Manduka eKO Mat ($76; manduka.com).

GIVE YOUR MAT A SECOND LIFE

You can double the feel-good benefits of your yoga practice without any extra sweat. Instead of trashing your old mat, donate it to Manduka's Recycle Your Mat program (recycleyourmat.com).

The company, which was founded by a yoga practitioner, will recycle, repurpose, or donate the mat, depending on its condition. As an added bonus: You'll score a 20 percent discount on Manduka products.

Visit their site for simple instructions on how to send in or drop off your old yoga mat.

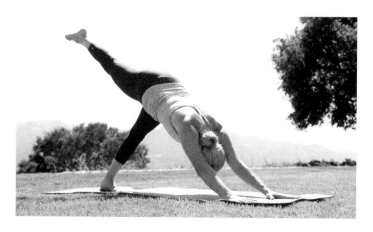

DOWN DOG CRUNCH
STRENGTHENS GLUTES AND CORE; STRETCHES BACK,
HAMSTRINGS AND CALVES

Start on your hands and knees, with your palms flat and slightly in front of your
shoulders, your knees under your hips, and your toes tucked under. Exhaling,
straighten your legs and press up into Downward-Facing Dog (your body should
resemble an inverted V), stretching your heels down toward the mat. Inhaling, lift
your right leg up, pressing your palms evenly into the mat.

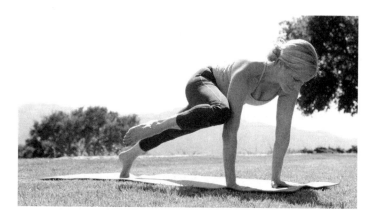

Exhaling, shift your torso forward into a plank position (keep your shoulders over
your wrists and your core engaged) and pull your right knee toward your right elbow.
Inhaling, reach your right leg back to the sky, returning to 1-legged Down Dog.
Do 10 reps. Switch sides and repeat.

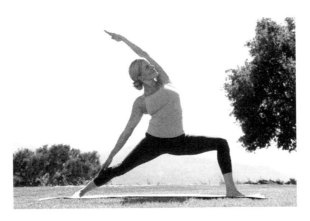

REVERSE WARRIOR TO SIDE ANGLE
STRENGTHENS GLUTES, THIGHS, AND CORE;
STRETCHES SIDE OF BODY

From Down Dog, step your left leg forward between your hands, bringing the side of your right foot parallel to the back edge of the mat. Inhaling, come into Warrior II, turning your hips and torso to the right and raising your arms to shoulder height, with your palms facing down. Flip your left palm up. Inhaling, come into Reverse Warrior, reaching your left arm up and leaning your torso back slightly, resting your right hand on your right leg.

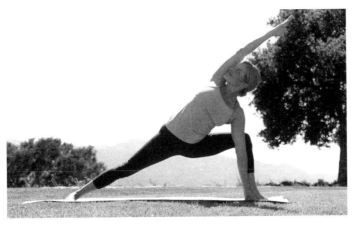

Exhaling, lean forward and rest your left forearm on your left thigh or beside your foot, reaching your right arm up and over your head, with your biceps by your ear, coming into a Side Angle Pose. Inhaling, come back to Reverse Warrior. Do 5 to 10 reps. Switch sides and repeat.

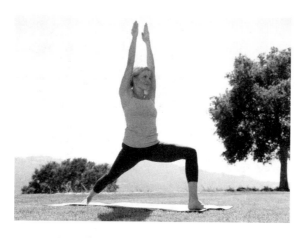

BOWING WARRIOR

STRENGTHENS GLUTES, THIGHS, AND CORE; STRETCHES SHOULDERS AND LOWER BACK

From Down Dog, step left foot between hands. Press right heel down and turn foot 45 degrees toward center of mat. Inhaling, come into Warrior I.

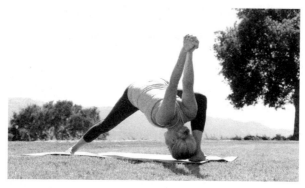

Interlace your fingers behind your back. Exhaling, fold forward, bringing your chest inside of your left thigh. Inhaling, lift back to the starting position, keeping your fingers interlaced. Do 5 to 10 reps. Switch sides and repeat.

(I DID IT!) ────────────────────────────────

"I wanted to feel healthier and develop a more positive body image, and this program helped me to do it. Plus, I dropped 10 pounds!"

—Carrie Barrepski

"I feel better physically, but I also feel better about myself. I have more definition in my arms and thighs, and I've lost 7 pounds."—Peggy Hughes

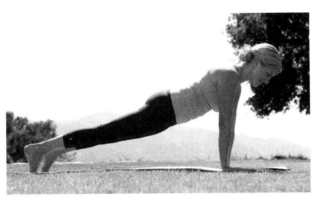

CHATURANGA PUSHUP
STRENGTHENS CORE, SHOULDERS, CHEST, BICEPS AND TRICEPS

Start in Down Dog. Draw your torso forward to a plank position, bringing your shoulders directly over your wrists and keeping your spine in one long line. Inhaling, engage your core and lengthen your spine, extending the crown of your head forward and pressing your heels back.

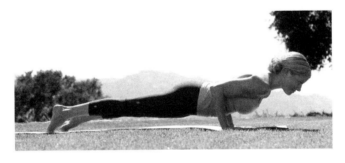

Exhaling, lower halfway to the mat, keeping your elbows close to your waist and your shoulders away from your ears. Inhaling, push back up to a plank position. Do 5 to 15 reps, gradually working up to 25.

Make it easier: Drop to your knees for Chaturanga Pushups, keeping your elbows pulled in and your shoulders away from your ears.

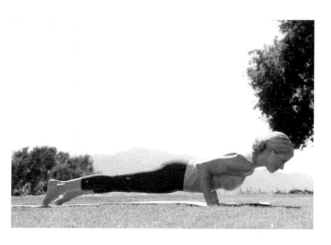

WARRIOR III CORE CRUNCH
STRENGTHENS GLUTES, LEGS AND CORE; STRETCHES HAMSTRINGS

Stand with your feet together in the middle of the mat. Inhaling, set your gaze on one point and contract your abs, shifting your weight onto your left leg. Exhaling, come into Warrior III, leaning your torso forward, hinging at your hips, and lifting your right leg off the mat and your arms out to the sides at shoulder height. (Your torso and right leg should be parallel with the mat.) Inhaling, lengthen through your arms and right leg.

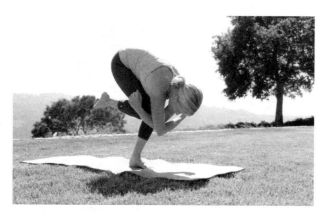

Exhaling, bend your left knee and crunch into a tight ball, hugging your arms to your chest, pulling your right knee toward your nose, and rounding your upper back. Inhaling, straighten your left leg and return to Warrior III, reaching your arms out to the sides and your right leg behind you. Do 5 to 15 reps. Switch sides and repeat.

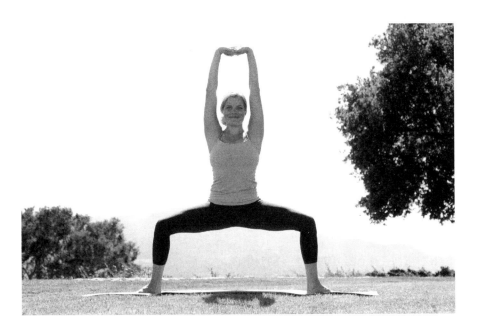

TEMPLE POSE

STRENGTHENS GLUTES, THIGHS AND BACK; STRETCHES UPPER
BACK AND SHOULDERS

Stand facing the long side of the mat, with your feet about 3½ feet apart and your
toes turned out. Tuck your pelvis under, aligning it with your spine (do not stick your
butt out), and engage your abs. Inhaling, interlace your fingers and press your arms
overhead. Exhaling, bend your knees about 90 degrees. Hold for 5 breaths. Inhaling,
straighten your legs halfway and repeat. Do at least 10 reps.

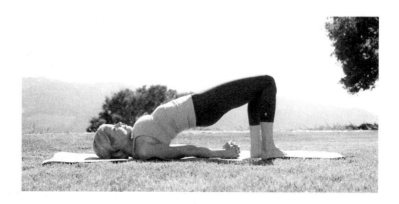

BRIDGE POSE WITH LEG LIFT
STRENGTHENS GLUTES AND THIGHS; STRETCHES SHOULDERS AND CHEST

Lie faceup on the mat, with your knees bent and hip-width apart, your feet flat on the mat and parallel, with your heels as close to your butt as possible. Inhaling, lift your hips off the mat. Clasp your hands below your pelvis and reach your fists toward your feet, rolling your shoulders underneath your chest, coming into Bridge Pose. Hold for 5 breaths, pressing your chest and hips up.

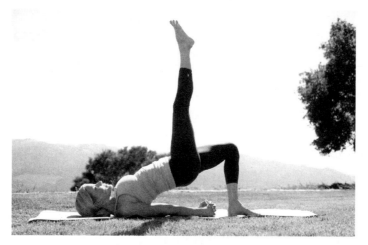

Continue to hold, or shift weight onto your left leg, and on an inhale, press through your left heel and lift your right leg straight up. Hold for 4 breaths. On an exhale, bring your right knee into your chest and release your foot to the mat. Inhale, then exhale, releasing your hips back down to the mat. Repeat the sequence on your opposite side to complete 1 rep. Do 2 or 3 reps.

JOY-BOOSTING JOURNALING

Journaling is an important part of this program because it helps release pent-up thoughts and emotions that contribute to negative behaviors.

"Many of us overeat due to emotional stress," Turner says. "Getting your feelings out will help you more clearly understand your relationship to food and your body. It also helps you tune in to your body and deepen your connection to your inner voice."

Do your Joy-Boosting Journaling assignment each week. To speed your progress, also do 10 to 15 minutes of free-form journaling each day. Simply write down whatever comes to mind. Don't edit yourself or hold back.

Week 1: Get to know your body. What's your long-term goal for your body? What do you want it to look like? More important, how do you want to feel in your body? Write down your plan to create the body that you want to live in.

Week 2: Fine-tune your desires. What would you do with your life if no one could criticize or praise you? How would you spend your time? Would your life be different? What does this tell you about how much power you give others? Write down your dreams and desires.

Week 3: Let go of past hurts. Is there someone who betrayed your heart or hurt you? Do you feel responsible for other people's burdens? What do you feel guilty about? What do you judge yourself for? Write it all out.

YOGA TURNS TEENS SWEET

If you've had enough of your teenager's foul mood and flippant attitude, take her with you to your next yoga class. According to a 2012 study published in the *Journal of Developmental & Behavioral Pediatrics*, after taking yoga two or three times a week for 10 weeks, 11th and 12th graders were less likely to feel anxious or in a bad mood than students who took a standard gym class.

"The slow, deep breathing used may help teens relax," says study author Jessica Noggle, PhD, a researcher at Harvard Medical School. "Yoga may also teach teens to look inside themselves instead of to their peers for acceptance and affirmation, which can help lower social stress and anxiety."

In Full Bloom

Everything's coming up roses—and petunias and poppies—for Valerie Bertinelli. Here, the star talks about the upside of getting older, her stay-slim secret weapons, her best beauty secrets, and why women rule the world.

You know you're in the presence of a serious exerciser when her first words to a visitor upon opening the door are "Come see my gym!" Ever-adorable Valerie Bertinelli, the 53-year-old dynamo with a new marriage and a buzzed-about hit TV show, *Hot in Cleveland*, has lots to be excited about, so if her home gym tops the list, we're curious.

The spare room in Bertinelli's new Los Angeles home houses his-and-her treadmills, an elliptical trainer, and a blue yoga mat with the signature logo of Jenny Craig, the weight loss program Bertinelli used to drop 40 pounds. On the wall is a flat-screen television, which is not used to watch goofy game shows or rival sitcoms while Bertinelli pounds away the pounds. It's a fat-shrinking tool.

"When I'm not motivated, I watch *Dancing with the Stars* or *The Biggest Loser*. They're working so hard, it makes me work harder," she says.

She then models her Walkvest, a 6-pound weighted vest she wears while on postdinner strolls around the neighborhood with hubby Tom Vitale. It helps boost her calorie burn, Bertinelli says. It also makes her look like the cutest SWAT team member ever.

With total aplomb, Bertinelli pops open a glucosamine-packed drink, Joint Juice. (She drinks it to protect her knees.) Then she leads the way to a cozy, book-lined study, where two leather armchairs face a window overlooking the San Fernando Valley. There she settles in to chat about her ongoing commitment to her health, why she's more confident than ever, and the unexpected challenges of a second marriage.

Prevention: Is it important for you to own being 53?

Bertinelli: I've been around so long I can't lie about it. It's an old cliché, but you really do get better as you age. I wish I had the body and the face of that 20 year old. I'm so glad I don't have her brain. I feel not necessarily smarter but more settled and informed than when I was that age. Everything was about "What do people think of me?" Now I'm calmer. Hopefully, I've gotten a little more grace.

Prevention: What didn't you like about yourself back then?

Bertinelli: I don't think I was a well-rounded human being. I was much more selfish. There's a fine line between taking care of yourself and not spoiling yourself. Do you know what I mean? Yet sometimes it's good to put yourself first, because then you have more energy to give to others. It's about finding balance.

Prevention: After six years together, you and Tom finally got married. Is your relationship different now?

Bertinelli: The relationship is the same, but it feels different. Making a commitment with our preacher and all our family there just means more. Something digs down deeper into your heart.

"Most days, I try to emphasize the good points and skip the bad ones."

Prevention: Does a second marriage present new issues?

Bertinelli: We have the old ghosts of our previous marriages that we have to work through. Certain words might trigger what he's heard in the past. My intention is not the same as his ex-wife's when she would say things to him, and vice versa—when he says something to me that sounds like an old ghost of mine.

"The only thing that makes me cranky is bad drivers."

Prevention: As a marriage veteran, why do you think men cheat?

Bertinelli: Why do women cheat? I don't know. It's a flaw in character. I had that flaw, and all it does is make you feel like crap. I never, ever want to feel that feeling again. It destroyed the trust between me and my first husband [musician Eddie Van Halen].

Prevention: Can people move beyond it?

Bertinelli: You can change. I know my ex-husband changed. I know that I've changed. Now I'm absolutely positive that if it gets so bad between me and my husband that we're not making a connection, then we'll break up before either one of us cheats, for the simple reason that I won't see that pain in another person's eyes again. I can't guarantee Tom won't cheat on me, but I'm pretty sure he won't.

Prevention: Do you think you would know if he did?

Bertinelli: You can talk yourself out of anything, even when all the signs are there, because you don't want them to be there, but I think now, I would know.

Prevention: Was it tough when your son, Wolfie, moved into his own place?

Bertinelli: I am so impressed with the way he lives his life. And his place is only a mile and a half from here. I can see it from one of my windows!

Prevention: Like so many women, you seem very centered. Why aren't women running the world?

Bertinelli: Well, maybe we are, but we let men think they're doing it because we live in a patriarchal society. In reality, I think we have a lot more to say than we let men know. But in a way, we do run the world. We're that soft shoulder for men to fall back on. I can totally see Michelle Obama, Laura Bush, or Hillary Clinton—all these great women who are married to presidents—running the world.

Prevention: You look just great. What's your workout these days?

"I like it when someone thinks I can do more even when I don't."

Bertinelli: I mix treadmill running with exercises such as pushups, walking lunges, crunches. Today I did my variation on a workout my trainer, Christopher [Ross Lane], gave me a long time ago that's always good in a pinch.

Prevention: Trainers are expensive. Is it worth cutting something out of your budget to get one?

Bertinelli: Absolutely. It's a really good investment. Health clubs all across the country have them. And you don't need one for any longer than one to two weeks. Get some good stuff, and write it down. Then do it on your own.

Prevention: You're at your target weight. What are some things you do to maintain it?

Bertinelli: If I know that I'm going to go out to dinner, I have a light, light breakfast and a light, light lunch, so I can indulge. It's more about portions. If I start restricting myself with any food, I'm going to obsess about it. Eventually I'll indulge, and I won't stop.

Prevention: Is it hard to get back on track if you slip and overeat?

"There's a fine line between taking care of yourself and not spoiling yourself."

Bertinelli: Sometimes I'll beat myself up for having too much, and then I'll go, okay, that's it. Did it, move on, be better next time.

Prevention: Do you have time to relax?

Bertinelli: I need to get a pedicure because this one's 3 weeks old. I'm trying to figure out how to do that, because there are other things I need to be doing—working out, laundry, painting, cleaning. With a massage, I only enjoy the first 10 minutes, and then the next 50 I'm like, okay, I have things to do.

Prevention: Do you have any bad beauty habits?

Bertinelli: I try not to forget to take my makeup off. I'll still pick at a pimple, and I know I shouldn't, but it's so tempting. Fifty-three, and you get pimples! How unfair is that? [laughs]

Prevention: Do you think about cosmetic surgery?

Bertinelli: Yeah. You see how the jowls start. Because of the business I'm in, you notice it more, but I haven't had work done. You can always tell when someone's had work. They don't quite look like themselves—cheekbones are a little bit higher. I'm not judging; we all want to feel better about ourselves. I don't want to look different from what people are used to. I look different enough by aging, but then to change my face trying for it not to age. You're never going to look like a 20 year old, so there's really no point. Of course, talk to me in 10 years and see, because this is starting to bug me, right here [pulls on her eyelids]. But I don't want my eyebrows to go up too much.

> *"You follow the Golden Rule, you're going to feel better."*

Prevention: How do you feel about something milder, like injectables?

Bertinelli: I'm curious about Botox, and I like the way some people look when they have it done right. I wouldn't mind getting rid of some of these lines here [points between her brows], but if I can't move them, I can't do comedy.

Prevention: Is there a rule you've learned to live by?

Bertinelli: Doing unto others as you would have them do unto you. There's nothing like it. You follow the Golden Rule, you're going to feel better. If you treat people the way you want to be treated, it's real simple.

GET VAL'S BODY—ONE DAY AT A TIME!

This simple workout should take only around ½ hour.

Set your treadmill at a 0.5 percent incline.

Walk for 2 to 3 minutes to warm up.

Walk at a fast pace for 8 minutes.

Do 30 crunches, 15 pushups, and 15 triceps dips.

Walk for 6 minutes.

Do 15 walking lunges on each leg and 30 squats.

Walk for 4 minutes.

Do 30 crunches, 15 pushups, and 15 triceps dips.

Walk for 2 minutes.

Do 15 walking lunges on each leg and 30 squats.

Perform two sets of 30 seconds of bicycle-kick abdominals (lying on back, lift shoulders slightly off floor, raise feet, and move legs in a pedaling motion for 30 seconds).

Stretch!

Note: On alternate days, instead of doing pushups, perform 15 biceps curls with dumbbells and 15 seated rows, using either a machine or bands.

Bonus Weight–Loss
RECIPES

On the pages that follow, you'll find *Prevention*'s best recipes to help you lose weight and look great. They're delicious, nutritious, and quick and easy, too.

PEAR TODDY

Achieve pear-fection by ripening this fabulous fruit at room temperature until the neck (or stem end) gives way to a little pressure. Pears are harvested while still hard (they get mealy if left to ripen on the tree), but they become soft, sweet, fragrant, and creamy in texture after a few days. Pears spoil quickly, so move them to the fridge once they're ripe.

Makes 2 servings

1 pear, peeled and chopped

1 teaspoon unsalted butter

2 cups apple cider

4" strip lemon peel

4" strip orange peel, plus more for garnish

¼ cup orange juice

1 tablespoon honey

4 cloves

1 cinnamon stick

¼ cup pear brandy

1 tablespoon fresh lemon juice

1. In a saucepan, cook the pear for 5 minutes in the butter over medium heat until softened. Add the cider, lemon peel, the 4" strip of orange peel, orange juice, honey, cloves, and cinnamon stick. Simmer for 10 minutes.

2. Through a sieve, strain the mixture into another saucepan. Stir in the brandy and lemon juice.

3. Pour into 2 mugs. Garnish with the remaining orange peel.

PER SERVING: 312 calories, 0 g protein, 55 g carbohydrates, 46 g sugars, 2 g total fat, 1 g saturated fat, 3 g fiber, 29 mg sodium

PICK THE PERFECT PEAR

Here are some of the delicious pear varieties you'll likely find at your local store.

ANJOU: **Better for eating**

BOSC: **Good for cooking and eating**

COMICE OR PACKHAM'S TRIUMPH: **Better for eating**

FORELLE: **Better for cooking**

PUMPKIN-BACON PANCAKES

These pancakes are a delicious treat for a lazy Saturday.

Makes 4 servings

½ cup whole wheat flour

½ cup all-purpose flour

¾ teaspoon baking powder

½ teaspoon pumpkin pie spice

¼ teaspoon baking soda

¼ teaspoon salt

¾ cup buttermilk

½ cup pumpkin puree

2 large eggs

2 tablespoons honey

1 tablespoon olive oil

2 strips cooked bacon, crumbled

¼ cup maple syrup

1. Preheat the oven to 200°F.

2. In a large bowl, whisk together the whole wheat flour, all-purpose flour, baking powder, pumpkin pie spice, baking soda, and salt.

3. In another bowl, whisk together the buttermilk, pumpkin puree, eggs, honey, and oil. Gently stir the buttermilk mixture into the flour mixture.

4. Preheat a cast-iron griddle coated with cooking spray over medium heat. In batches, drop heaping tablespoonfuls of the batter onto the griddle to form 3" pancakes (about 12). Cook for 2 minutes, or until the bottoms are golden. Sprinkle with the bacon. Flip and cook for 2 minutes, or until the bottoms are golden.

5. Finish cooking and keep warm in the oven for 5 minutes. Drizzle with the syrup.

PER SERVING: 304 calories, 10 g protein, 50 g carbohydrates, 25 g sugars, 8 g total fat, 2 g saturated fat, 3 g fiber, 442 mg sodium

SEEDS FOR SOUNDER SLEEP

Whether you're cooking or carving a pumpkin, be sure to save the seeds, which pack magnesium, a mineral that might ward off migraines and improve sleep. Swish the seeds in water to separate them from the pulp. Drain, then spread on an oiled pan. Dry for 10 minutes at 350°F, stirring once. Toss with oil and seasonings. Bake for 10 to 15 minutes, stirring, until golden.

SAUSAGE-STUFFED MUSHROOMS

These fantastic fungi bring meaty texture and complex flavor to dishes for very few calories.

Makes 8 servings

24 small white mushrooms (about 1 pound)

3 ounces hot Italian pork sausage

¼ cup panko bread crumbs

Small basil leaves for garnish

1. Preheat the oven to 400°F.

2. Remove the stems from the mushrooms and arrange the mushrooms on a baking sheet. Finely chop half of the stems.

3. In a medium bowl, stir together the stems, sausage, and bread crumbs. Mound into the mushroom caps.

4. Bake for 20 minutes, until cooked through. Garnish with the basil.

PER SERVING: 56 calories, 3 g protein, 3 g carbohydrates, 1 g sugars, 4 g total fat, 1 g saturated fat, 1 g fiber, 86 mg sodium

GRILLED VEGETABLE PASTA SALAD

You could mix it up by trying different vegetables in this pasta salad.

Makes 6 servings

½ pound baby zucchini, halved

½ pound eggplant, cut into ⅓"-thick rounds

½ pound red onions, cut into ¼"-thick slices

¼ teaspoon salt, divided

¼ teaspoon ground black pepper, divided

½ pound cellentani or rotini pasta

½ cup basil pesto

3 tablespoons sliced, dry-packed sun-dried tomatoes

3 tablespoons pine nuts, toasted

1. Prepare a lightly oiled grill for medium heat (or use grill pan).

2. Coat the zucchini, eggplant, and onions on both sides with olive oil spray, and season with ⅛ teaspoon of the salt and ⅛ teaspoon of the pepper. Grill the vegetables (in batches if necessary) for 6 minutes, turning, until golden brown and tender. Transfer the vegetables to a cutting board and cut into bite-size pieces.

3. In a large pot of boiling water, cook the pasta according to the package directions. Drain and immediately toss in a serving bowl with the pesto, tomatoes, and grilled vegetables. Season with the remaining ⅛ teaspoon of the salt and ⅛ teaspoon of the pepper. Sprinkle with the pine nuts.

PER SERVING: 283 calories, 8 g protein, 39 g carbohydrates, 7 g sugars, 11 g total fat, 1 g saturated fat, 6 g fiber, 321 mg sodium

MUSHROOM PIZZAS

Avoid mushrooms with dark or wet spots or a mildewy smell. Store mushrooms in their original packaging (put loose ones in a paper bag) and refrigerate for 3 to 4 days. Rinse them gently and pat dry, or wipe with a damp paper towel, just before using. But never soak them. Because they're so porous, they'll become waterlogged.

Makes 4 servings

4 small portobello mushroom caps (8 ounces total)

6 tablespoons marinara sauce

4 tablespoons shredded part-skim mozzarella cheese

2 teaspoons basil pesto

1. Preheat the oven to 425°F.

2. On a baking sheet, place the mushroom caps gill side down. Roast for 20 minutes.

3. Flip over and fill each cap with 1½ tablespoons of the marinara sauce and 1 tablespoon of the cheese.

4. Bake for 2 minutes, or until the cheese is melted and the mushrooms are tender.

5. Top each with a dollop of basil pesto.

PER SERVING: 61 calories, 4 g protein, 5 g carbohydrates, 1 g sugars, 3 g total fat, 1 g saturated fat, 1 g fiber, 160 mg sodium

GRILLED CHICKEN WITH MANGO MOJO

Gently squeeze mangos to judge ripeness. A little give means it's ready to eat.
(The color of the skin isn't an accurate indicator.) A sour odor (or loose, wrinkly skin)
is a tip-off that the fruit is past its prime and mushy.

Makes 4 servings

1 mango, peeled, pitted, and chopped

3 tablespoons lime juice

3 tablespoons finely chopped jalapeño peppers without seeds

3 tablespoons finely chopped cilantro

1 teaspoon minced garlic

1 teaspoon ground cumin

1¼ pounds chicken breasts

1 teaspoon olive oil

¼ teaspoon salt

¼ teaspoon ground black pepper

1 lime, cut into wedges

1. In a blender, puree the mango and lime juice.

2. Transfer the mango mixture to a bowl and stir in the jalapeño peppers, cilantro, garlic, and cumin.

3. Brush the chicken with the oil and sprinkle with the salt, jalapeño, and black pepper. Grill the chicken on a lightly oiled grill over medium heat for 12 minutes, turning once, until the chicken is cooked through. Serve with mango mojo and the lime wedges.

PER SERVING: 261 calories, 37 g protein, 14 g carbohydrates, 12 g sugars, 6 g total fat, 1 g saturated fat, 2 g fiber, 350 mg sodium

STEAK, PEPPERS, AND MASHED POTATOES

This hearty family-friendly dish comes together in around half an hour.

Makes 4 servings

1 pound russet potatoes, peeled and cut into 1" chunks

1 pound cauliflower florets

½ cup low-fat buttermilk

¼ teaspoon salt, divided

¼ teaspoon ground black pepper, divided

1 pound trimmed flank steak

3 cloves garlic, minced

1 pound mini sweet peppers (12–18 total)

1 tablespoon balsamic vinegar (optional)

1. In a large saucepan, cover the potatoes and cauliflower with 2" of cold water. Bring to a boil. Simmer for 15 minutes, until tender. Drain and return to the pan. Mash with the buttermilk and season with ⅛ teaspoon of the salt and ⅛ teaspoon of the pepper. Cover and keep warm.

2. Preheat the broiler while the vegetables cook. Rub the top of the steak with the garlic and sprinkle with the remaining ⅛ teaspoon of the salt and the remaining ⅛ teaspoon of the pepper. Place on one side of a foil-lined sheet pan. Arrange the sweet peppers on the other side of the pan. Lightly coat all with olive oil spray. Broil 6" from the heat for 10 minutes, turning, until the peppers are golden brown on both sides and the steak is cooked to medium-rare. Remove the steak to a cutting board.

3. Let the steak rest for 10 minutes before slicing. Spoon the mashed potatoes onto plates and serve with the steak and peppers. Drizzle the peppers with the vinegar, if using.

PER SERVING: 321 calories, 31 g protein, 35 g carbohydrates, 8 grams sugars, 7 g total fat, 3 g saturated fat, 6 g fiber, 311 mg sodium

MANGO-SHRIMP RICE NOODLES

Keep unripe mangoes on the counter until they soften slightly.
Put them in a paper bag to speed the process.

Makes 4 servings

4 ounces medium-thick rice noodles

2 scallions, sliced

6 tablespoons lime juice

¼ cup cilantro leaves

4 teaspoons sesame oil

2 teaspoons honey

1½ teaspoons finely grated ginger

¾ pound cooked shrimp, halved

1 large carrot, cut into matchsticks

1 cup cucumber, cut into matchsticks

1 mango, peeled and chopped

1. In a pot of boiling water, prepare the noodles according to the package directions.

2. In a large bowl, stir together the scallions, juice, cilantro, oil, honey, and ginger.

3. Add the drained noodles, shrimp, carrots, cucumber, and mango. Toss.

PER SERVING: 326 calories, 22 g protein, 46 g carbohydrates, 17 g sugars, 6 g total fat, 1 g saturated fat, 4 g fiber, 829 mg sodium

PISTACHIO CLOUDS WITH FRESH FRUIT

This elegant dessert is impressive yet easy to prepare. Pistachios supply heart-healthy fats and cholesterol-lowering phytosterols. The antioxidants in raspberries and the potassium in citrus fruits help keep blood pressure under control.

Makes 2 servings

2 tablespoons finely chopped natural pistachios

2 tablespoons confectioners' sugar

2 large egg whites

¼ teaspoon cream of tartar

¼ cup granulated sugar

½ cup raspberries

¼ cup clementine or seeded tangerine segments

1 teaspoon chopped fresh mint leaves

1. Preheat the oven to 250°F. Line a baking sheet with parchment paper.

2. In a small bowl, toss the nuts with the confectioners' sugar. Set aside.

3. In a separate bowl, beat the egg whites with the cream of tartar with an electric mixer at high speed for 1 minute, until soft peaks form. Gradually add the granulated sugar with the mixer running and beat for 1 minute, just until stiff peaks form. Gently fold in the nut mixture.

4. Drop the mixture in 2 mounds, 5" apart, on the prepared pan. With a spoon, make a 2½"-diameter bowl in the center of each mound. Use a spatula to smooth the edges to form approximately 5"-diameter rounds.

5. Bake in the center of the oven for 1 hour, until dry and crisp on the outside. Transfer the parchment paper to a rack and cool the meringues completely. (Store them in an airtight container in a cool, dry place until ready to serve.)

5. In a bowl, mix the raspberries, clementine, and mint. Place the meringues on 2 serving plates and fill with the fruit mixture. Serve immediately.

PER SERVING: 214 calories, 6 g protein, 42 g carbohydrates, 37 g sugars, 4 g total fat, 1 g saturated fat, 3 g fiber, 56 mg sodium

BAKED MAPLE PEARS

Pears and other white-fleshed fruit might help protect against stroke, according to a recent Dutch study.

Makes 4 servings

4 firm, ripe medium pears

⅓ cup maple syrup

2 tablespoons sanding (coarse) sugar

4 quarter-size slices ginger

1 star anise

1. Preheat the oven to 375°F.

2. Trim the bottoms of the pears. Stand the pears upright in a baking dish that's just large enough to hold them. Drizzle the pears with the syrup. Sprinkle the sides of the pears with the sugar. Add the ginger and star anise to the baking dish.

3. Tent the pears with foil and bake for 50 minutes, until tender. Discard the star anise. Drizzle the pears with the syrup mixture remaining in the baking dish.

PER SERVING: 224 calories, 1 g protein, 59 g carbohydrates, 46 g sugars, 1 g total fat, 0 g saturated fat, 7 g fiber, 6 mg sodium

Part 3

FITNESS
MOVES

133

CHAPTER 12

SLIM + SCULPT STRAPS ROUTINE

Go from frumpy to fit in 5 fast weeks with our best-ever walking-and-toning workout. Your new secret weapon: suspension straps!

Are you showing up for your sweat sessions but not seeing results?

Your equipment might need an upgrade. Enter: suspension straps, the one-piece-does-it-all Swiss Army knife of fitness gear. Loved by personal trainers, these versatile nylon straps hook to any stable anchor, such as your bedroom door or a sturdy tree branch, and they allow you to use your own body weight as resistance. They require minimal space, weigh only about 2 pounds, and can be stashed in a drawer between uses. You can even tuck them into a suitcase for on-the-road workouts. They're also fun to use, and you can control how challenging each move is. Bonus: Because strap moves require balance, they engage your core muscles, flattening your belly fast.

What's more, our Slim + Sculpt Straps routine (see page 137), created by *Prevention* contributing editor and personal trainer Chris Freytag, will slim

Aim to do three Slim + Sculpt Straps sessions and three or four 20- to 30-minute Cardio Walk sessions each week. Feel free to swap days according to your schedule.

DAY 1	DAY 2	DAY 3	DAY 4	DAY 5	DAY 6	DAY 7
Slim + Sculpt Straps	Cardio Walk 20 minutes	Slim + Sculpt Straps	Rest	Cardio Walk 30 minutes	Slim + Sculpt Straps AND Cardio Walk 20 minutes	Cardio Walk 30 minutes

you from head to toe in only 20 minutes a day, 3 times a week! We had real women test the plan using the Jungle Gym XT suspension system ($99; lifeline-usa.com). To melt fat faster, they also squeezed in three or four quickie Cardio Walks (see below) each week and followed a 1,600-calorie diet. After 5 weeks, the numbers on the scale plummeted. The women's average weight loss was more than 8 pounds, and one tester even dropped a whopping 18.6 pounds—for some women, that's three whole sizes—as well as 10 inches total off her waist, hips, and thighs!

CARDIO WALKS

You don't have to work out for hours on end to burn off unwanted jiggle. Simply do 20 to 30 minutes of brisk walking at an intensity at which you're breathing hard but can still speak in short sentences. Do cardio walking on the same day as your strap circuit for a longer, fat-blasting workout or on alternate days when you're pressed for time.

Your total workout time should be 20 to 30 minutes.

How to do it: Start with a 2-minute warmup of slow walking (or walking in place). Do 2 sets of 15 reps of each exercise, resting for no more than 30 seconds between sets and when adjusting straps before moving to the next exercise. (The fast pace keeps your heart rate elevated, which boosts calorie burn.) To protect your back and maintain balance, be sure to keep your abs engaged and your head in line with your spine throughout each move. End with a 2-minute cooldown of full-body stretching.

Your total workout time should be 20 minutes.

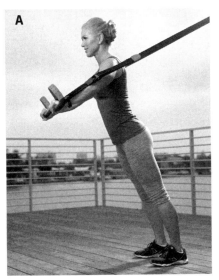 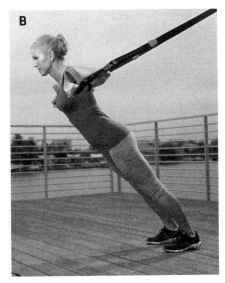

CHEST PRESS

TARGETS CHEST, ARMS, AND CORE

Anchor your straps. Stand facing away from the anchor point, with your feet hip-width apart and your arms extended slightly lower than chest level and holding the handles (A).

Leaning into the handles, slowly lower as if doing a pushup (B).
Return to the starting position and repeat.

Boost your burn: Begin with your body positioned at a steeper angle to increase the resistance.

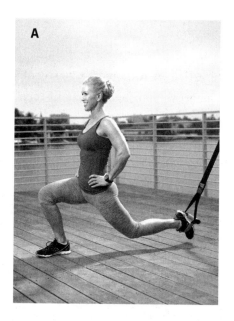

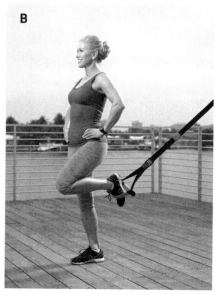

FOOT-UP LUNGE
TARGETS THIGHS, GLUTES, AND CORE

Stand facing away from the anchor point, with your left foot in the cradle of 1 strap. Bend your right knee into a lunge, lowering your left knee toward the ground (A).

Slowly stand, pulling your left foot toward your right shin (B). Return to the starting position. Do 15 reps on each leg to complete 1 set.

Make it easier: Hold on to a chair for extra balance.

YES, YOU CAN BE TOO THIN

A 5-foot-4 woman who weighs 160 pounds might be healthier and live longer than one who tips the scales at 100, says William D. Lassek, MD, coauthor of *Why Women Need Fat*. Yes, being obese is unhealthy, but just a little extra weight gives you more infection-fighting white blood cells without raising your other risks too high.

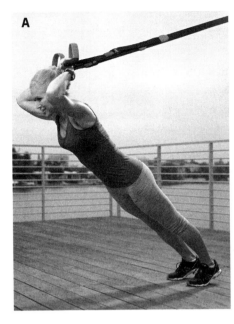

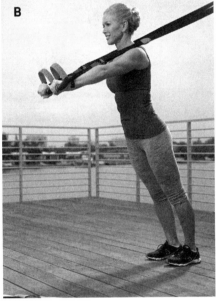

TRICEPS PRESS
TARGETS TRICEPS AND CORE

Stand facing away from the anchor point, with your feet hip-width apart and your arms at your sides, holding the handles. Raise your arms, bending your elbows and bringing your biceps near your ears, leaning your body forward (A).

Extend your arms to chest level, raising your body to almost standing straight (B). Return to the starting position and repeat.

"I'm not very coordinated, but the straps are still working! They're changing my entire body, not just single muscle groups!"

—Joni Heinsch lost 18.6 pounds

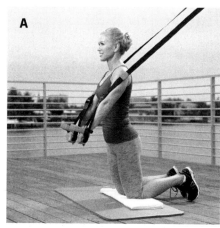

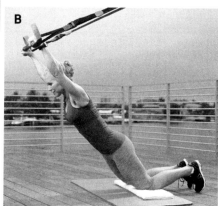

KNEELING BODY ROLL-OUT

TARGETS ARMS AND CORE

Place a folded towel under your knees for extra padding. Kneel facing away from the anchor point, with your arms extended toward the ground a few inches in front of you, holding one handle in each hand (A).

Lean into the handles and slowly raise your arms overhead, lowering your torso toward the ground (B). Return to the starting position and repeat.

A 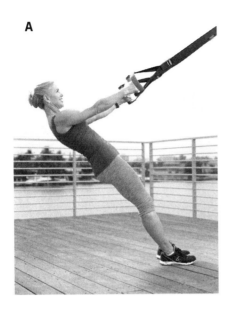 **B**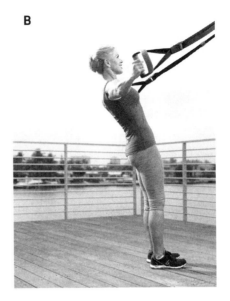

REAR DELTOID FLY
TARGETS BACK, ARMS, AND CORE

Facing the anchor point and holding the handles with your arms extended, lean back until the straps are taut (A).

Pull your chest forward, using your upper back to extend your arms out to the sides (B). Return to the starting position and repeat.

Make it easier: Bend your elbows as you extend your arms out to the sides.

"My posture is improving, and I no longer have that hunched-over feeling!"

—Trudi Detert lost 6.6 pounds

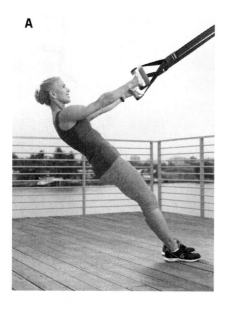

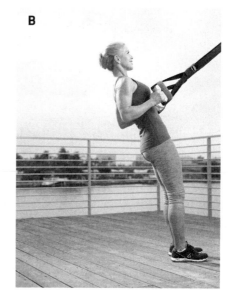

BODY ROW
TARGETS ARMS, BACK, AND CORE

Stand facing the anchor point, holding one handle in each hand with your arms extended. Lean back until the straps are taut (A).

Pull your chest forward, bending your elbows and squeezing your shoulder blades, bringing your hands alongside your chest until you are almost standing straight (B). Return to the starting position and repeat.

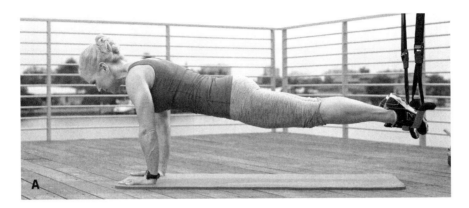

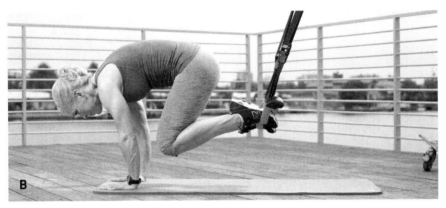

KNEES TO ELBOWS
TARGETS CHEST AND CORE

Starting on all fours, hook your toes into the strap cradles. Walk your hands forward into a plank pose (A).

Slowly pull your knees toward your elbows, engaging your core and lifting your hips skyward (B). Return to the plank position and repeat.

Make it easier: Instead of pulling your knees toward your elbows, rest your weight on your forearms and hold a static plank pose for 30 seconds.

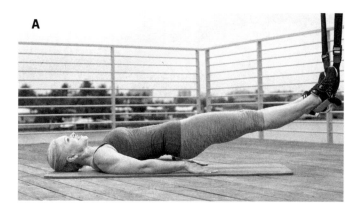

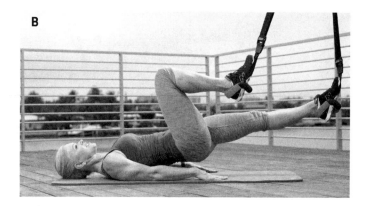

RUNNER
TARGETS GLUTES, HAMSTRINGS, AND CORE

Lie faceup on the ground, with your heels in the foot cradles under the anchor point and your arms extended at your sides. Pressing through your glutes, lift your lower back a few inches off of the floor (A).

Pull your right heel toward your glutes, keeping your left leg extended (B). Switch legs, drawing your left heel toward your glutes and extending your right leg. Keeping your hips raised, continue alternating legs for 30 seconds to complete 1 set.

YOUR NEW TRIM-DOWN TOOL

The 7½-foot nylon straps on the Jungle Gym XT safely support your weight when anchored to a solid three-hinged door or any sturdy beam, tree branch, or pole. They allow you to use your own body as resistance in more than 100 different exercises—all without making a trip to the gym or junking up your living room with bulky fitness equipment!

Here's how to use them once they're secured.

1. Press down on the tab to slide the cam buckles up and down the strap to adjust length.

2. Hold on to the handles to do everything from pushups to triceps extensions.

3. Tuck your feet into the foot cradles for exercises such as single-leg lunges and suspended plank poses.

CHAPTER 13

A FLATTER BELLY— AT ANY AGE

Stay strong and slim through your forties, fifties, and sixties by following this science-backed plan.

If a genie gave you the chance to change one thing about your body, what would you wish for? If you'd ask for a flatter belly, you've got plenty of company— 72 percent of women ages 45 to 64 named the abs the body part they felt most insecure about, according to a recent survey by the research firm Mintel.

It's no wonder. The more birthday candles you blow out, the more difficult it is to keep belly fat at bay. In your youth, estrogen surges encourage your body to store protective fat in the hips and buttocks to prepare for pregnancy. As estrogen levels begin dropping in your forties and fifties, lower-body fat pulls up stakes and resettles right where you don't want it: on your stomach.

"The body stores fat in the belly because it can access and use that fat quickly for energy, which was critical hundreds of years ago, when the body was fine-tuned for periods of starvation," says Marie Savard, MD, a women's health physician in Philadelphia and the author of *The Body Shape Solution to Weight Loss and Wellness*.

147

Here's another belly inflator: "Starting around age 30, sedentary women lose 5 to 7 pounds of muscle every decade," says Wayne Westcott, PhD, a *Prevention* advisory board member and director of fitness research at Quincy College in Massachusetts. "This lowers your metabolic rate by 2 to 4 percent every 10 years, causing you to slowly pack on weight even if you're not eating more calories."

A bigger belly affects your wardrobe, and it also sets you up for health problems. Underneath the subcutaneous fat (the muffin top you can grab with your hand) lies more-harmful visceral fat, which builds up around your organs and pushes against your abdominal wall.

"Visceral fat produces chemicals that create harmful inflammation in the body, increasing your risk of heart disease, diabetes, and even cancer," says Scott Isaacs, MD, a clinical instructor of medicine at Emory University School of Medicine in Atlanta and the author of *Hormonal Balance*. The good news: Whittling your waist a mere 2 inches is enough to take you out of the danger zone.

Follow our plan for a strong, slim, and healthy middle in your forties, fifties, and sixties. Each decade builds on the one before, so you'll have an arsenal of strategies by the time you reach your sixties. Starting the plan midway? Review the other decades and build to where you need to be. You could see results in as few as 2 weeks!

YOUR FORTIES

Your abs now: There's a good chance that you're starting to notice a little extra belly flab. That's because as you begin perimenopause, estrogen levels start to drop, and your metabolism dips too if you don't exercise regularly. Stress might also contribute, because tension triggers the release of the hormone cortisol, which causes your body to store more visceral fat.

Big-Belly Health Risks

Low bone density: A bigger-than-ideal belly puts you at greater risk of osteoporosis, according to a study in the journal *Bone*.

THE 10-POUND ADVANTAGE

D on't interpret this as permission to park yourself on the couch or visit the drive-through daily, but being a little overweight might not be such a bad thing, especially when you're older. After evaluating data from more than 9,000 adults ages 70 to 75, researchers found that overweight individuals (those who had a BMI of 25 to 29.9) had the lowest mortality rate—13 percent lower, in fact, than normal-weight individuals.

"Being overweight when you're older might provide a nutritional reserve or buffer when you get sick," says study coauthor Leon Flicker, PhD, of the Western Australian Centre for Health and Ageing.

"High visceral fat is associated with decreased levels of growth hormone and insulin-like growth factor 1, which are both important for bone health," says Miriam A. Bredella, MD, lead study author and assistant professor of radiology at Harvard Medical School.

Best Belly-Flattening Strategies

Make protein a priority. Protein helps prevent muscle loss, so to stem the depletion and keep your metabolism humming, shoot for 0.45 grams of protein per pound of body weight daily, says Christine Gerbstadt, MD, RD, the author of *Doctor's Detox Diet.* If you weigh 140 pounds, that's about 63 grams.

Kick up your cardio. High-intensity interval training (HIIT) is best at blasting belly fat. Research has shown that women who did 20 minutes of HIIT 3 times a week burned more fat than women who exercised at a moderate pace for 40 minutes 3 times a week. To reap the benefits, progress to 25 minutes of HIIT 3 to 6 days a week. Alternate between 2 to 3 minutes at a challenging pace and 1 minute at a moderate pace.

Shrink your waist with weights. To slow muscle loss, tone your major muscle groups 2 or 3 times a week. Start by performing 1 to 3 sets of 8 to 12 repetitions of each exercise, using 8- to 15-pound dumbbells.

Limit libations. Nobody's saying you have to be a teetotaler, but too much alcohol stimulates cortisol production, Dr. Isaacs says. Limit servings and try to avoid beer because of its belly-fat-building carbohydrates.

Your Best-Belly Moves

The following powerful planks strengthen the core and fight muscle loss, which begins to cause belly rounding in this decade. You'll also tighten muscles that might have been stretched during pregnancy. Do 3 sets of each move 2 or 3 times a week.

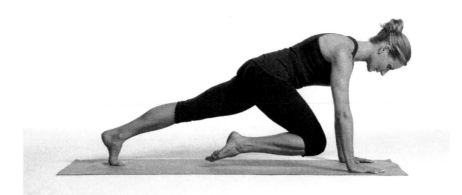

MOUNTAIN CLIMBER

Start in a pushup position, with your wrists under your shoulders. Contracting your abdominals, bring your right knee toward your chest. Repeat on the opposite side to complete 1 rep. Do 10 reps.

HOW MUCH BELLY FAT IS TOO MUCH?

You don't need to see a doctor to know if you have too much abdominal fat. Just pull out a tape measure and wrap it around your waist. If the result is under 35 inches (under 40 inches for a man), give yourself a clean bill of belly health.

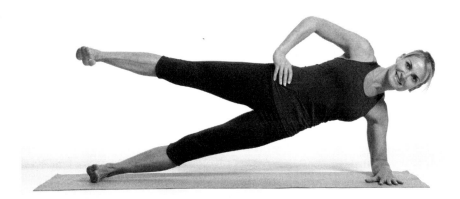

FOREARM SIDE PLANK

Lie on your left side, with your elbow in line with your shoulder and your feet stacked. Contracting your abdominals, lift your hips so that your body forms one long line. Lift your right leg and hold for 10 seconds. Do 3 reps on each side.

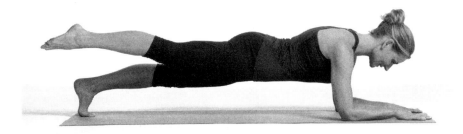

PLANK REACH

Start in the plank position. Raise your right arm in front of you. Lower; repeat with your left arm. Lower; lift your right leg off of the floor. Lower; repeat with your left leg to complete 1 rep. Do 3 reps.

YOUR FIFTIES

Your abs now: The big drop in estrogen during menopause makes your midsection become rounder. In fact, within the first few years after menopause, women gain about 10 pounds, most of which goes straight to the waistline. Plus, "the decrease in sex hormones results in more easily disturbed sleep for many women," says Lisa Shives, MD, founder of Northshore Sleep Medicine in Evanston, Illinois. Besides making you more tired, lack of sleep causes hormone imbalances that can increase your appetite.

Big-Belly Health Risks

Insulin resistance: As you move into your fifties, you're at greater risk of developing insulin resistance, a condition that causes the body to produce more insulin than it should, Dr. Isaacs says. The excess causes you to store more fat and increases your appetite. The double whammy: Too much belly fat further ups your risk of insulin resistance, which can lead to diabetes.

Best Belly-Flattening Strategies

Wipe out wheat. "One slice of whole wheat bread increases blood sugar more than 1 tablespoon of sugar does," says William Davis, MD, a preventive cardiologist in Milwaukee and the author of *Wheat Belly*. That blast of sugar prompts your body to release insulin, setting the stage for increased storage of visceral

SLIM YOUR BELLY, BRIGHTEN YOUR MOOD

Parting with a little belly blubber is only good for your health and confidence, and it can also give you a mental boost.

"Clients often tell me that they feel happier after losing weight," says Vonda Wright, MD, an orthopedic surgeon in Pittsburgh.

Here are two possible reasons: Exercise stimulates feel-good hormones that can last up to 12 hours, and the healthier you are, the less sick you are, which allows you to be more productive.

fat. When you remove wheat from your diet, your appetite drops dramatically, and you begin losing belly fat, Dr. Davis says.

Pump up protein. To offset age-related muscle loss, increase protein in your diet as you age, Dr. Gerbstadt says. In your fifties, shoot for 0.5 gram for every pound of body weight. A 140-pound woman should consume 70 grams daily.

Be smart about sleep. With your hormones working against you now, it's more imperative than ever to develop proper sleep hygiene, which includes keeping your bedroom cool and dark, as well as banishing anyone—snoring husbands or pets—who might disturb you.

Fine-tune your fitness. Have a few more aches? Swap 2 of the HIIT walks you did in your forties with moderate-paced walks, logging at least 5 sweat sessions weekly. To guard against metabolism-slowing muscle loss, continue to do 2 strength workouts each week.

Your Best-Belly Moves

The following moves tighten abs, prevent further belly rounding caused by reduced muscle mass, and challenge balance, which decreases as you age. Do 3 sets of each move 2 or 3 times a week.

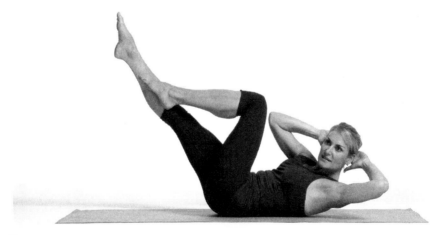

BICYCLE CRUNCH

Lie on your back, with your knees over your hips. Lift your shoulder blades off of the floor. Drive your right elbow toward your left knee while extending your right leg. Switch sides to complete 1 rep. Do 12 to 16 reps.

REVERSE CRUNCH

Lie on your back, with your legs extended upward directly over your hips. Contracting your abdominals, lift your hips a few inches off of the floor. Slowly lower your hips, then your legs, toward the floor. Do 8 to 12 reps.

ELEVATED TREE POSE

Step your left foot on top of a yoga block. Contract your abdominals and place your right foot on your left inner calf. Extend your arms overhead. Hold for 10 breaths. Switch sides and repeat.

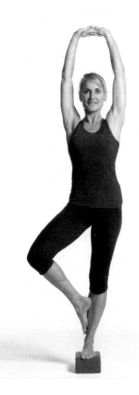

YOUR SIXTIES

Your abs now: Although your estrogen levels might be the same as they were in your fifties, you're still losing muscle due to aging. That further slows your metabolism, which is why belly fat continues to be an issue. Osteoporosis could also be making your tummy appear rounder.

"As you lose bone mass, you become shorter," Dr. Savard says. Because there's no place for your organs to go, your abdomen protrudes.

Big-Belly Health Risks

Increased inflammation: While the extra candles on your birthday cake are cause for celebration, in this decade, belly fat might trigger greater amounts of inflammation in your body, further increasing your risks of heart disease and diabetes.

Knee pain: Too much weight around your belly puts extra stress on your joints, often leading to knee pain that can limit activity.

Best Belly-Flattening Strategies

Keep your sneakers handy. Just as you did in your fifties, continue to walk at least 5 days a week, aiming for 2 or 3 HIIT power walks and 2 longer, moderate strolls. If you're having trouble increasing your pace, hit the hills to get your heart pumping.

Stay strong. In your sixties, strength training becomes even more crucial for keeping your metabolism humming, as well as for maintaining bone density. Just don't switch to wimpy weights.

"You might need to reduce the weight slightly, but it shouldn't be significant," says Irene Lewis-McCormick, IDEA fitness expert and a personal trainer in Des Moines, Iowa.

Be a hottie. Regular yoga will strengthen your core, but if you can tolerate it, try hot yoga, which is done in a heated studio. As you age, "collagen breakdown makes belly skin look saggy, even if you have good muscle tone," Lewis-McCormick says. "Hot yoga releases toxins, which helps maintain skin elasticity."

Add a protein power snack. Make one more adjustment to your protein needs, increasing to 0.55 grams per pound of body weight. A 140-pound woman should consume around 77 grams daily.

Your Best-Belly Moves

The following moves challenge balance and zero in on the foundation of a solid core, the transverse abdominis, which is a muscle women often lose awareness of as they age. Do these moves 2 or 3 times a week.

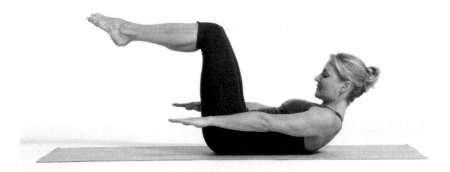

HUNDRED

Lie on your back with your knees over your hips, and your arms by your sides. Lift your shoulders off of the floor. Take 5 breaths in through your nose and 5 out through your mouth, pumping your arms. Repeat 10 times.

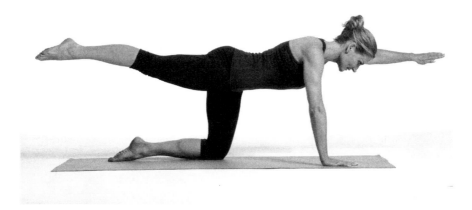

QUADRUPED BALANCE

Start on all fours. Extend your left arm in front of you to ear height and your right leg behind you to hip height. Hold for 5 to 8 seconds. Switch sides to complete 1 rep. Do 8 reps.

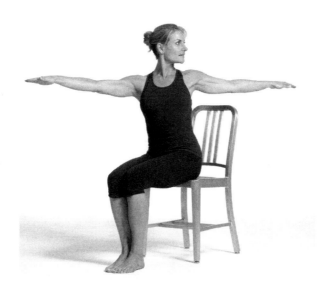

SEATED SPINAL TWIST

Sit in a chair and extend your arms out at your sides. Exhale and twist your torso halfway to your left. Inhale, then exhale again, twisting as far as you can. Repeat to your right to complete 1 rep. Do 20 reps.

CHAPTER 14

YOUR SUPERFAST INDOOR WORKOUT

Is it too hot? Too cold? Too rainy? That's no excuse! You can keep your workouts inside with the following routine that trims, tones, and burns off stress—in minutes!

Our secret for preventing weight gain inside, at home, is multitasking body-weight moves that combine cardio and strength training for a metabolism-revving workout that you can do anywhere. You don't need weights, bands, straps—nada, just yourself.

"Incorporating exercises that require multiple muscles boosts heart rate and burns more calories in less time," says Jarett Perelmutter, owner and head trainer at Brick Sport Performance Training in Los Angeles and the creator of this routine.

Do each move for 1 minute. Without sacrificing form, complete as many reps as possible. Rest for 20 seconds after each exercise. If you're up for the challenge, perform the entire circuit 3 or 4 times.

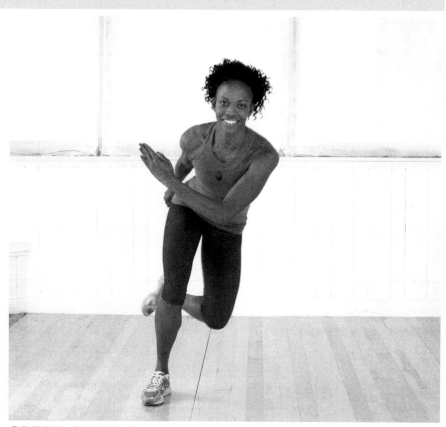

SPEED SKATER
TARGETS BUTT AND THIGHS

Stand with your feet hip-width apart, with your arms by your sides. Hop to the right, landing on your right foot while sweeping your left foot diagonally behind your right leg and swinging your left arm across your body and your right arm behind your back. Jump to the left, switching your legs and arms to complete 1 rep.

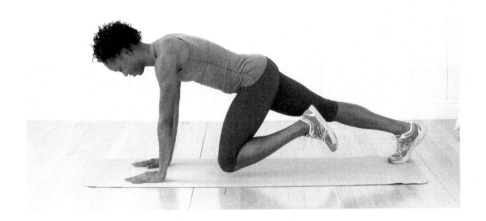

MOUNTAIN CLIMBER
TARGETS ABS, SHOULDERS, BACK, AND BUTT

Begin in a plank position, with your wrists directly under your shoulders and your body in a straight line from your head to your ankles. Keeping your upper body still, bring your left knee toward your chest. Return your left leg to the starting position while simultaneously bringing your right knee forward, as though jogging. Continue alternating legs.

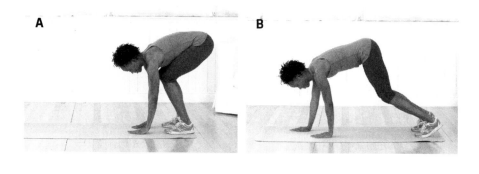

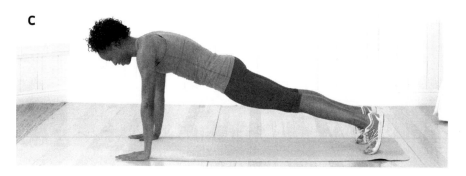

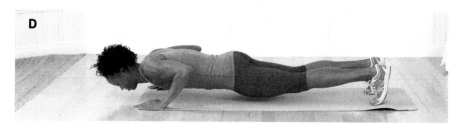

INCHWORM WITH PUSHUP
TARGETS ABS, ARMS, SHOULDERS, CHEST, AND BACK

Stand with your feet hip-width apart. Fold forward, bringing your palms to the floor (bend your knees if necessary) (A). Walk your hands forward (B) to a plank position, with your wrists under your shoulders (C). Perform 1 pushup (D) (modify by bringing your knees to the floor if needed). Walk your hands back to your feet; stand up to complete 1 rep.

A

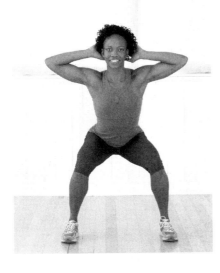

B

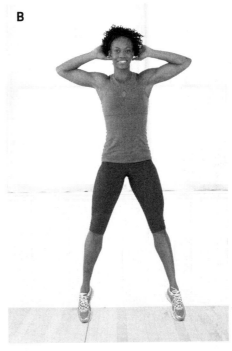

SQUAT JUMP
TARGETS BUTT AND THIGHS

Stand with your feet slightly more than hip-width apart, your hands behind your head, and your elbows out. Squat, pushing your hips back and bending at your knees; keep your chest upright and your knees behind your toes (A).

Push off of the floor and jump as high as possible (B), immediately lowering into the next squat.

CHAPTER 15

THE WALKING WORKOUT

You can stand sideways — with confidence! The following walking workout — no dieting required — will melt off up to 5 inches and 13 pounds from your figure in just 4 weeks!

Bored with your walking routine? Pump up the fun and the fat burn with this 50-minute interval routine created by Lee Scott, a walking coach and the owner of Wow Power Walking in Toronto.

Walking is the foundation of the workout. You'll walk to warm up, cool down, and recover from the hard effort of the intervals. But it's the cardio and strength-training drills (the hard halves of the intervals) that will really help sculpt your body and blast extra calories. Because these 10 moves focus on your core, you'll see a big change in your abs.

Scott trained 12 women using this program 4 times a week, and in just a month, one lost 5 inches off her waist! The 11 others had similarly excellent results, losing inches and pounds while gaining tone and definition.

THE WORKOUT AT A GLANCE

Do this 50-minute workout 4 times a week. The moves and format will stay the same throughout, but starting in week 3, you'll do longer cardio and strength intervals. Going harder for longer will boost your muscular and cardiovascular endurance.

Your total workout time is 50 minutes, consisting of:

WARMUP: **10 minutes: Walk at an easy to moderate pace: 5 minutes. Walk at a brisk pace: 5 minutes.**

CARDIO INTERVALS: **10 minutes: Alternate cardio intervals ("hard") with walking ("recover"). During recoveries, walk as fast as you can while still allowing your breath to slow. (See page 167.)**

STRENGTH INTERVALS: **20 minutes: Alternate strength intervals ("hard") with walking ("recover"). During recoveries, walk as fast as you can while still allowing your breath to slow.**

COOLDOWN: **10 minutes: Walk, moving from a brisk pace to a moderate to easy pace for 7 minutes, and then stretch your calves, quads, and hamstrings for 3 minutes.**

WEEKS 1 AND 2: **Do each cardio interval exercise for 30 seconds, then recover for 30 seconds. Complete the circuit twice, for a total of 10 minutes.**

Do each strength interval exercise for 30 seconds, then recover for 30 seconds. Complete the circuit 4 times, for a total of 20 minutes.

WEEKS 3 AND 4: **Do each cardio interval exercise for 60 seconds, then recover for 60 seconds. Do the circuit once, for a total of 10 minutes.**

Do each strength interval exercise for 60 seconds, then recover for 60 seconds. Complete the circuit 2 times, for a total of 20 minutes.

CARDIO INTERVALS

After you've warmed up for 10 minutes, it's time for 10 minutes of cardio intervals. Do each of the following moves in the order described for 30 or 60 seconds, per the guidelines on page 166.

Skip: Hop on your left leg while bending your right knee up to hip height. Travel forward, alternating sides.

Walk

Side Shuffle: Stand with your knees bent in a half squat. Shuffle to the left 4 times, hopping as your legs come together. Stop, then shuffle to the right 4 times. Alternate sides.

Walk

Lunge with Twist: Step forward with your left foot into a lunge. Twist your torso to the right. Step your right foot to meet your left. Alternate sides, moving forward.

Walk

Lateral Hop: With your hands on your hips and your feet together, hop to the left 12 to 24 inches, then to the right 12 to 24 inches. Repeat.

Walk

Curb Climb: Step up onto a curb or stair with your left foot, then your right foot. Step down. Repeat, alternating sides.

Walk

After your cardio, it's time for 20 mintues of strength training. Alternate the following strength moves with walking, following the time guidelines on page 166. These moves are the "hard" part of the interval; walking is the "recover" portion.

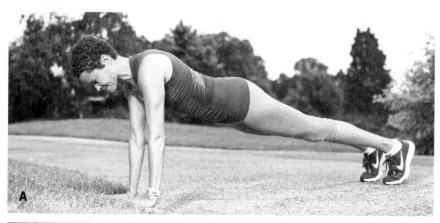

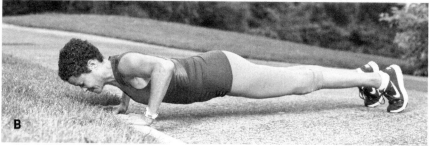

PUSHUP

Start in a plank position, with the balls of your feet and your palms on the ground, and your hands slightly more than shoulder-width apart (A). Bend your elbows wide, bringing your body toward the ground. Straighten your elbows to push your body up (B).

Make it easier: Place your hands on a bench or wall and do pushups with your upper body higher than your lower body.

Make it harder: Lift one leg as you do pushups. Do three pushups with your right leg lifted, then three with your left leg lifted. Continue alternating sides.

A

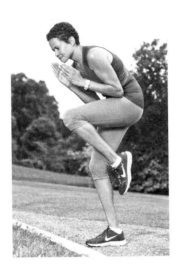

B

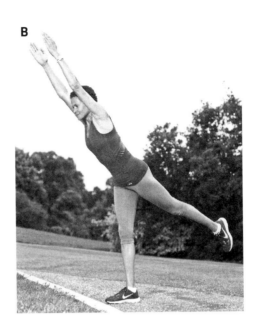

STANDING BIRD DOG

Stand on your right leg with your left knee bent toward your chest and your arms at your sides, with your elbows bent (A). Extend your left leg back and reach your arms overhead (B). Your torso and left leg should be extended about 45 degrees from vertical. Hold for 1 second, and then return to the starting position. Do this on your left for 1 interval, and then switch sides for the next interval.

Make it easier: Extend your leg only, keeping your hands on your hips.
Make it harder: Extend your leg and torso parallel to the ground.

"I usually walk twice a week, but I needed a boost after having a baby. This program was great!"
—Julie Grinbergs lost 5 pounds and trimmed 4 inches
off her belly in 4 weeks

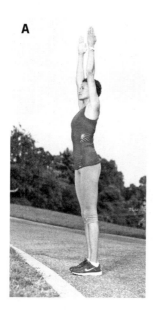
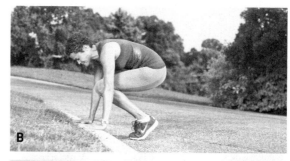
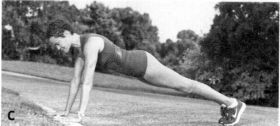

BURPEE

Stand with your arms reaching overhead, with your feet together (A). Squat low, bringing your hands to the ground just outside of your feet (B). Quickly jump back with both feet to a plank position (C). Jump forward again to a low squat. Stand up, extending your arms overhead.

Make it easier: Step one leg at a time to the plank position and then step forward to a squat.

Make it harder: Add a pushup each time you're in the plank position.

"Usually I work out with a buddy, but this program was easy to do on my own—the time flew, and I didn't get bored."

—Anne Gibson lost 2½ inches off her belly in 4 weeks

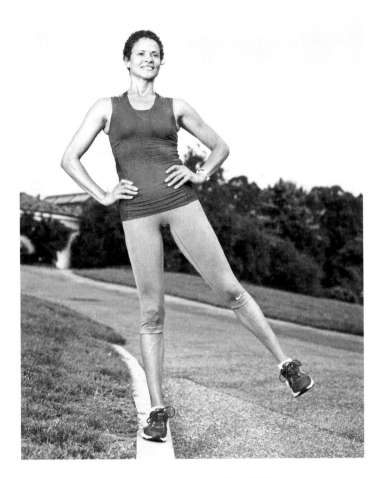

CURB SQUAT WITH SIDE LEG PRESS

Stand with your right foot on top of a curb and your left foot next to the curb, on lower ground. Press into your right foot and straighten your right leg. Extend your left leg out to the side, with your left knee and toes facing front. Lower to the starting position; that's 1 rep. Do it on the same side for 1 interval, and then switch legs for the next interval.

Make it easier: Do it on level ground. Skip the squat and simply lift your leg to the side.

Make it harder: Do not touch down while extending your leg between repetitions. Keep all of your weight on your standing leg for the duration of the interval.

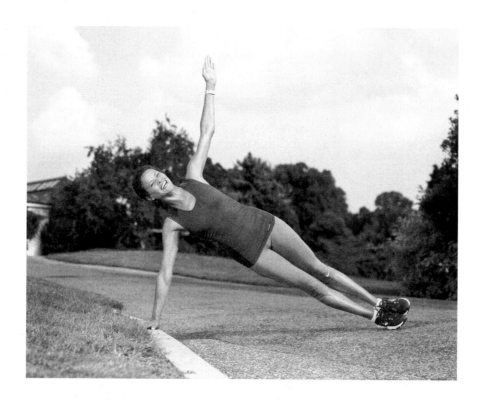

SIDE PLANK

Balance on your right hand and the outside edge of your right foot so your body is in a straight line from your head to your heels, with your shoulders, hips, and legs off the ground. Extend your left arm upward. Hold for the duration of the interval. Alternate sides for each interval.

Make it easier: Rest your forearm or knee on the ground.

Make it harder: Lift your top leg 6 inches off of your bottom leg, so your top leg is hovering in the air.

COOL DOWN

After completing the circuit, cool down for 10 minutes.

INTERVALS MADE EASY

Here's how to use your favorite gadget to make your workout easier.

IF YOU HAVE A SPORTS WATCH: Use the interval function. Most watches can be set to beep each time a certain number of seconds pass.

IF YOU HAVE A SMARTPHONE: Download the free app Gymboss Interval Timer (itunes.apple.com). Customize your interval length; it will sound a tone when it's time to move to the next exercise.

IF YOU HAVE A WATCH WITH A SECOND HAND: Walk for half the length of a single interval, make note of how far you've gone, and then double back to your starting spot—that's your 30- or 60-second walk, which you'll repeat. Use your watch to time the cardio and strength moves.

"I liked that there are different levels for each move. I could really tell when I was getting stronger."

—Missy Westgate lost 5 inches off her belly in 4 weeks

CHAPTER 16

OUR ULTIMATE GREAT HEALTH GIFT GUIDE

From steals to splurges, here are good-for-you gifts to inspire you and everyone on your list to slim down, shape up, get fit, stress less, and feel great!

Winter, spring, summer, or fall, no matter what the season, you can find a reason to splurge on someone you love. If you need more justification, why not buy something for someone you love to help them be healthier and happier? Here are some great ideas to gift to practically anyone.

GIFTS FOR THE CARDIO JUNKIE

The runners and bikers on your list will love these finds.

Fashionably fit: The slim-fitting Under Armour StudioLux Noir Jacket

($148; ua.com) is the haute couture of the fitness world. Fashion-forward details make this moisture-wicking performance jacket a must-have.

Cool drinker: The BPA–free CamelBak Eddy Glass Water Bottle ($25; camelbak.com) offers 25 ounces of stylish hydration. Bonus: The removable silicon sleeve protects it from breaking if tossed around in a gym bag.

DIY personal trainer: The Gymboss Interval Timer ($20; gymboss.com) makes interval and circuit training a breeze. It programs up to 99 intervals and beeps between sets.

Savvy traveler: On-the-go exercisers will love the compartment for stinky

SMARTER FITNESS FOOTWEAR

Want to get more out of your favorite workout classes such as Zumba and aqua aerobics? Treat your feet to a pair of shoes made specifically for the demands of each.

BEST FOR DANCE CARDIO: Unlike regular sneakers, the Reebok Urlead ($75; reebok.com) has a traction-free "spin spot" located under the ball of each foot to help you twist and pivot without sticking to the floor. Plus, extra cushioning helps reduce shock during jumps, keeping your feet comfy.

BEST FOR WATER AEROBICS: Make a splash at your next aqua workout with Speedo Hydro Comfort 2.0 ($65; speedousa.com). The rubber bottom grips the pool floor, ensuring you feel surefooted and powerful. Bonus: The ventilated mesh upper allows water to drain easily, so shoes dry faster postworkout.

BEST FOR PILATES: Keep sweaty feet steady when sculpting on the Reformer machine with Blake Brody in-Studio Footwear ($98; blakebrody.com). Traction pads prevent slipping off the foot bar, and the comfy, flexible soles allow natural, barefootlike movement.

BEST FOR BARRE: Trust the shoemaker of choice for prima ballerinas. Capezio's Fizzion ($40; capezio.com) is customizable with straps and laces to guarantee a snug, supportive fit. Another pro: The grippy sole offers extra control (without sticking) when balancing.

sneakers in Lug's Puddle Jumper Wheelie Bag ($170; luglife.com). It's ventilated so odors can escape.

Charming words: Commemorate a fitness feat with the Heart 13.1 fitness charm necklace ($78; ericasaradesigns.com). You can inscribe a message on the back at no extra cost.

Muscle saver: Train hard, recover smart. Magnesium sulfate and essential oils in Soak bath crystals ($5 for 7 ounces; soakfitness.com) fight muscle fatigue postworkout.

Cleanup act: Say sayonara to sweat stains with Roux Maison Sport Laundry Detergent ($17; rouxmaison.com). The gentle formula helps workout wear last longer.

Pedal power: Giro's Petra cycling shoes ($80; giro.com) give Spinning classes a shot of energy with a fun pop of teal. Plus, the antimicrobial foot bed combats odor.

FOR THE YOGA LOVER

If you have any yoga devotees on your list, they'll appreciate these thoughtful gifts.

Divine power: No-slip grips on Yogitoes Deity Continuum rSkidless Yoga Towel ($64; yogitoes.com) stabilize footing, and the Hindu deity designs add a spiritual touch.

Made-to-order mats: Surprise a special yogi with an Aspen Yoga Mat ($60; aspenyogamats.com) created just for her. Choose from 25 colors and designs for the perfect combo.

Germ fighter: Jo-Sha Wipes ($13 for 20; joshawipes.com) use toxin-free essential oils such as eucalyptus and lavender to de-grime mats, and they smell divine too.

Eco-friendly assist: Modify and correct alignment in poses with the biodegradable, toxin-free Manduka Bamboo Block ($25; manduka.com). It's Earth-friendly and pretty!

(continued on page 180)

TAKE A HIKE!

Here we pick the best boots to weather any trail.

BEST FOR STEEP SLOPES: Adidas AX 1 Mid GTX: Lace up these high-traction boots to handle intimidating elevation changes with ease. The stabilizing mid-cut top keeps feet in place, so you're less likely to twist an ankle. ($135; adidas.com)

BEST FOR BACKPACKING: Vasque Talus WP: Built for intrepid explorers, these boots have durable, cushioned soles that can support the weight of a backpack (up to 40 pounds). ($150; backcountry.com)

BEST FOR STREET-TO-TRAIL WEAR: Asics GEL-Scout: They might look like trendy sneakers, but they're trail-ready. A plastic plate protects feet from rocks, and wide-set lugs boost traction in mud. ($120; asics.com)

BEST FOR ALL-DAY LIGHT HIKES: Ahnu Montara 2: A great pick for trekking beginner to intermediate trails, these supportive low-cut hikers keep feet extra comfortable and blister free even on sunrise-to-sundown excursions. ($130; ahnu.com)

BEST FOR MUDDY/WET TRAILS: The North Face Havoc Mid GTX XCR: Muddy conditions are no threat, thanks to the easy-to-clean leather toe and wraparound mudguard. Plus, the high-stitched tongue helps keep water out. ($160; thenorthface.com)

BEST FOR TRAIL-RUNNING INTERVALS: Merrell Mix Master Glide: Rev your calorie burn by breaking into a jog in these versatile hikers. The low heel offers solid grounding without sacrificing grip. ($100; merrell.com)

GET THE BEST FIT

To find your perfect pair of hikers, keep in mind these suggestions from Sam Mackey, REI footwear specialist.

BE SMART ABOUT SOCKS. Socks affect the fit of a boot, so shop with a well-used pair you'll wear on the trail. The snug feel of new socks might make you decide a well-fitting boot is too tight.

PUT 'EM TO THE TEST. Do a few laps around the store. If anything pinches or rubs, keep shopping.

TIME YOUR TRY-ON. Shop midafternoon to early evening, when feet are their largest.

PAIR THEM WITH THE RIGHT SOCKS

Wear the wrong sock and even the best hiking boot will leave you begging for a chair. The following four get the nod for innovation and comfort, on and off the trail.

FOR EXTRA ENERGY: Goodhew Sockwell Women's Circulator: Graduated compression zones fight fatigue. ($25; goodhew.us.com for retailers)

FOR ODOR CONTROL: Sierra West Madras: Antimicrobial bamboo yarn prevents stinky feet. ($14; walkingcompany.com)

FOR COOL COMFORT: Keen Targhee Lite Crew: Moisture-wicking merino wool keeps temps in check. ($16; keenfootwear.com)

FOR BLISTER PROTECTION: Asics Trail Shield Quarter: Silicone traction pads keep feet in place, reducing painful rubbing. ($16; asics.com)

Handy helper: Colorful Gaiam Yoga Mat Bands ($5 each; amazon.com) keep mats neatly rolled between stretch sessions—and make great stocking stuffers.

Sweet savasana: Baked Ideas' funky Yoga Cookie Cutters ($32.50 per set; bakedideas.com) make cute and delicious gingerbread cookies (recipe included) worthy of sharing.

Tee-rific: The light and airy Lucy Prana Yama Burnout Tee ($59; lucy.com) looks lovely during class or while running errands after.

Zipped-up Zen: The Hotdog Rollpack Yoga Mat Bag ($90; hotdogyoga.com) has a garment compartment for hanging apparel so it doesn't wrinkle, plus extra storage spots for everyday necessities.

Luxe leggings: The plush fabric of Beyond Yoga Quilted Long Leggings ($82; beyondyoga.com) feels soft against skin, and the chic pattern slims thighs.

FOR THE ADVENTURE SEEKER

Skiers, hikers, and more will adore these ideas.

Feeling shady: Oakley's protective Elevate Snow Goggles ($150; oakley.com) are every ski bunny's dream. The face-conforming design ensures all-day comfort, and the antifog lens boosts visibility while protecting eyes from 100 percent of UV rays.

Core control: Keep your favorite outdoor exerciser cozy in subzero temps with the Columbia electro amp Core Vest ($150; columbia.com). Its battery-powered heating system creates a cocoon of warmth for hours, making it the ideal winter layer.

All-weather warrior: Slip a pair of Kahtoola Microspikes ($60; kahtoola .com) over shoes or boots to prevent falls during icy walks or runs. Metal teeth give feet a confidence-boosting grip.

Snow queen: Wind, rain, snow: The Isis Diva Jacket ($325; isisforwomen .com) can brave it all, thanks to its waterproof shell and the insulating, sweat-wicking fabric.

Foot buddy: Fashion meets function in these Teva Lenawee WP Boots ($170; teva.com). The waterproof shell keeps tootsies dry, and hard-core traction steadies feet.

Cool stepping: Engineered for a woman's foot, Tubbs Xplore Snowshoes ($130; tubbssnowshoes.com) turn any snowy terrain into a spot for calorie-torching adventure.

Lovely layers: Forget bulky thermals. Icebreaker Sprite Leggings and Racerback Bra ($70, $50; icebreaker.com) are made of thin merino wool for a no-itch, breathable fit.

Sweet snack: Stay fueled for action with tasty and convenient all-natural Barre energy bars ($2.50 each; realfoodbarre.com). Our fave is the Pirouette Cinnamon Pecan.

FOR THE AT-HOME EXERCISER

Gift your family and friends who work out at home with these great products.

DJ on demand: Stick the OrigAudio Rock-It 3.0 Speaker ($35; origaudio .com) to any object (coffee mug, cabinet) and plug it into a music source to fill any room with sound.

Soul soother: Invigorate workouts with the uplifting grapefruit scent of the SoulCycle by Jonathan Adler candle ($42; soul-cycle.com). Light, sniff, and sweat!

Sweaty sidekick: The New Balance N4 Lime ($70; nbmonitors.com) heart-rate monitor makes it easy to track calories burned, motivating exercisers to push harder.

Burn booster: Wrap Moore Trainer Resistance Bands ($90; mooretrainer .com) just above knees to add a fun challenge to lower-body moves such as squats and lunges.

Three-way recovery: Give tight, sore muscles a little extra TLC after challenging sweat sessions with the space-saving Gold's Gym 3-in-1 Massage Roll ($30; Walmart).

Best in bells: Empowers 3-in-1 Kettlebell ($40; empowerfitness.com) adjusts to 5, 8, or 12 pounds. Its plastic shell is easier on floors than traditional iron bells.

Hood happy: The classic hoodie gets a modern makeover with the sleek Adidas Modern Classics Grete Long Sleeve Hoodie ($45; adidas.com). The moisture-wicking fabric keeps skin comfy, cool, and dry.

Waist cincher: Mix and match weighted and nonweighted segments of Empower's Cardio Core & More Hoop ($40; empowerfitness.com) to create three heart-pumping—and totally fun—belly-firming workouts. Bonus: It breaks apart, so it's travel-friendly!

FOR THE HAPPY WALKER

Put a little spring in your family's and friend's steps with these great ideas.

Flash forward: Brooks' Nightlife Essential Run Jacket II ($85; brooks running.com) is what every runner wants: a slim-fitting, lightweight, windproof, water-resistant jacket with sleek reflective details.

Pole perfection: Stability-increasing, shock-absorbing REI Traverse Shock-light Women's Trekking Poles ($79.50; rei.com) boost calorie burn and add an upper-body workout to any walk.

Fit fingers: Touchscreen-friendly pads on the North Face Etip Gloves ($45; thenorthface.com) allow multitaskers to change songs and answer calls, keeping digits warm.

Pony perfect: Moving Comfort's Foxie Beanie ($18; movingcomfort.com) accommodates a ponytail, and sweat-wicking fabric keeps heads warm and dry.

Buff cuffs: Removable weights in W8Fit Cuffs (cuffs $19, weights $5; w8fit .com) add a little extra resistance to walks, sculpting arms and increasing calorie burn.

Hearing aid: These updated Apple EarPods ($29; apple.com) are designed to fit comfortably inside ears, so they won't fall out midworkout.

Stat tracker: Stay motivated with a Fitbit Zip pedometer ($60; fitbit.com). It tracks steps taken, distance traveled, and calories burned. Plus, it logs progress online.

Cozy cutie: Stay warm during walks with a chunky-knit Grayson Scarf by Pistil ($40; athleta.com). It's the perfect antidote to drab, chilly weather.

BRAIN BOOSTERS

Give the gift of improved memory, alertness, and concentration with the following science-backed picks.

Looking for a challenge beyond Sudoku or crossword puzzles? Try a tactile 3-D brainteaser, such as this Wooden Cube Puzzle ($5; scientificsonline.com).

The scent of rosemary, which wafts from the Izola Rosemary Candle ($35; izola .com), can significantly improve memory and make you feel more alert.

Certain audio signals played in stereo, featured on Hemi-Sync CDs ($20; hemi-sync.com), unite the brain's left and right hemispheres for better concentration, according to company-run research.

Give in to your next chocolate craving: Types containing at least 70 percent cacao, such as Fearless Chocolate ($6; fearlesschocolate.com), might stave off dementia.

The presence of indoor plants, such as the UncommonGoods Succulent Wall Planter Kit ($100; uncommongoods.com), could improve cognitive performance, say researchers in Norway.

Chewing Think Gum ($2; thinkgum.com), which contains caffeine, peppermint, and ginkgo biloba, improves aspects of memory, according to research published in the journal *Appetite*.

40 IS BETTER THAN 30

At the beginning of her best decade ever, Brooke Burke-Charvet has a lot to say about beauty, breast health, Botox, and more.

"I like improvising. When things go wrong, you can make them work, and great moments are created. It's thrilling; it's exciting; it's adrenaline." Brooke Burke-Charvet is talking about the rush she gets on *Dancing with the Stars*, the live megahit she has cohosted (oh, those fit-like-a-glove gowns!) since 2010, 2 years after she won the celebrity dance contest's glittering Mirror Ball Trophy. But embracing whatever life throws at her is clearly how the 42-year-old prefers it.

Not all the challenges of her life have occurred at work. She took an emotional risk when she ended her marriage to plastic surgeon Garth Fisher in 2005. By then, the couple had two daughters, Neriah and Sierra. Burke-Charvet found love again, however, with an old flame, former *Baywatch* star David Charvet. After having two children together—daughter Rain and son Shaya—they married in 2011.

Now Burke-Charvet is more likely to be found toggling between car pools and conference calls for one of her two online businesses—product site Babooshbaby.com and advice portal ModernMom.com. We sat down for a chat.

Prevention: **How do you keep in shape?**

Burke-Charvet: I spend as little time as I possibly can to get the best results—5 days a week if I'm lucky, or a minimum of 3. I'll do my own DVD. It's a 55-minute body-sculpting workout that's old-school moves—squats, side lunges, dips, kicks—that we made more dynamic. You use multiple body parts and move at a pace where you also get cardio benefits. I go to a Pilates Plus class once or twice a week. Today, I went to the gym and did 20 minutes of cardio. That's all the time I had.

Prevention: **What's your cardio workout?**

Burke-Charvet: Treadmill on a 15 percent incline at 3.5 mph. My heart rate's in the right zone to burn fat, get a good sweat. I'll be on a conference call, watch TV, or listen to music. Sometimes I don't listen to anything. I like that half hour of peace.

Prevention: You've publicly nixed tabloid rumors that you had a tummy tuck. What's the secret to your great core?

Burke-Charvet: Posture has a lot to do with it—keeping your core engaged, whether you're sitting, driving, or working at your computer. I've always done ab work, even when I was pregnant.

"To me, 'prevention' means being brave enough to be aware. It takes time, but I want to be around to take care of my family."

Prevention: Have you had a mammogram yet?

Burke-Charvet: Yes. As soon as I found out that my friend Giuliana Rancic [*E! News* anchor and *Fashion Police* cohost] was diagnosed with breast cancer, I booked my mammogram. I called her from the doctor's office and said, "Thank you for provoking me to have this done."

Prevention: **What was your experience like?**

Burke-Charvet: When I was finished, I said to the nurse, "What's the big deal? There's so much negative talk about the mammogram." The biggest thing was scheduling my day to get there. The actual appointment was a piece of cake.

Prevention: **You've talked about having melasma, which is a facial skin discoloration that often comes on during pregnancy.**

Burke-Charvet: Yes, and I'm like that one in 1,000 cases where it didn't go away after childbirth. I went to the best doctors. I did all the peels. I'm hoping hormonally, I'll roll out of it. I use CellCeuticals SPF 55+ sunscreen, and I never lie out in the sun, which really stinks, because I'm a sun girl.

Prevention: **Any other health concerns?**

Burke-Charvet: I have Hashimoto's, which means my thyroid doesn't function. I take a synthetic thyroid pill. I don't even like to take an aspirin, but I have to take this every day.

Prevention: **What does "prevention" mean to you?**

Burke-Charvet: It's being brave enough to be aware. David and I recently spent a day doing all our medical work. I had a 3-hour physical. It's a pain in the butt, but I want to be here to take care of my family.

Prevention: **You've been very candid about having breast enhancements in your twenties. Have you thought of having them redone?**

"After my first mammogram, I said to the nurse, 'What's the big deal?' The hardest part was scheduling my day to get there."

Burke-Charvet: I have. When you've breast-fed four children, things kind of change. So that's probably the most likely thing on the radar. I went through a phase where I wanted to have smaller breasts. Sometimes it's easier in dresses and gowns.

Prevention: **Have you had any other procedures?**

Burke-Charvet: I've done little bits of Botox for a long time. If I wasn't on TV, I probably wouldn't. Fillers at a minimal level are okay, but it scares me because I don't want to have that bloated look. In our industry, people do too much too soon or just too much. There's nothing worse than that frozen "I'm 40 but I want to look 25" look.

Prevention: **Your ex-husband was the first surgeon selected to appear on** *Extreme Makeover.* **Did he ever give you advice about plastic surgery?**

Burke-Charvet: He said, "Do as little as you have to do." I'm so lucky. He's like, "Please don't ever do any of that. It scares me." I'll just be happy and wrinkled instead.

Prevention: **Did you have any anxiety about turning 40?**

Burke-Charvet: Forty is better than 30. I have a better understanding of who I am, what makes me tick, what's okay and not okay. I've had such a great experience professionally in the past 3 to 4 years that it really opened my eyes to not procrastinating.

"As they get older, women get more comfortable in their skin."

Prevention: **Have you had a moment when you felt older?**

Burke-Charvet: I was hosting the Miss America pageant, and I was having a great time. Then it hit me: I could be any one of these girls' mothers! That's when I realized

I'm freaking 40. It was weird.

Prevention: **Young girls face so many obstacles to having a positive body image. How do you help your daughters overcome those roadblocks?**

Burke-Charvet: I would never put on a pair of jeans that were too tight and say, "I feel so fat today" in front of my girls. Words like those affect them.

Prevention: **Have any of your kids had an issue with weight?**

Burke-Charvet: At her last checkup, the pediatrician told my middle daughter that if she didn't get more exercise and eat less carbs, she could become...he might have used the word obese.

Prevention: **So what did you do?**

Burke-Charvet: I had a conversation with her, but I tried not to make it about weight. She asked, "Mommy, do you think I'm fat?" I said, "No. I think you're beautiful. I want you to be healthy just like I want your brother and sisters to be healthy." It's a delicate situation when raising girls. You can't weigh them or totally deprive them, or it plants the seed for a lot of issues.

"I spend as little time working out as I possibly can to get the best results. Today, I did 20 minutes of cardio. It was all the time I had."

Part 4

NUTRITION
NEWS

CHAPTER 17

WHAT DOCTORS REALLY EAT

What's on the menu for the nation's top doctors? Tasneem Bahatia, MD, asked dozens of them and got some healthy—and delicious—answers.

As a physician, I'm used to my patients asking, "What would you do if you were me?" when we're discussing treatment options. Over the past few years, though, they've begun making additional inquiries: What do you do to stay healthy? Do you eat fat? Sugar? Do you cook?" They see me as someone who has a lifestyle similar to theirs, with a family and a demanding job, but who also has insider knowledge of what really works (and what doesn't).

That's why I teamed up with the editors of *Prevention*. I realized that people want to learn more from their doctors—not only what science has found to be effective but what they do in their own lives. We contacted 64 health professionals and asked them for their best tips and recipes. The result is an incredible collection of advice from some of the nation's top experts.

I was initially set on my own path to nutritional awareness after becoming frustrated with my own health. As a medical student, I had limited understanding of nutrition. I was swayed by the "fat-free" craze of the '80s, so I loaded up on carbs and avoided fatty foods. I exercised aggressively and didn't concern myself with calories, protein, or healthy fats. Honestly, I didn't even know that I needed to worry about those things.

I patted myself on the back when I had popcorn for dinner or a green salad with fat-free dressing for lunch. I stayed away from junk food and fried food, so I thought I was a healthy eater. Between work and family demands, I was on a stress roller coaster, but I continued to try to sustain myself on low-calorie, low-fat foods.

Fast-forward a few years to when the "payback" began. At the age of 28, I battled weight gain, acne, and hormonal irregularities. My hair, which was once my crowning glory, started coming out in chunks. I actually had bald patches!

Around that time, I became interested in traditional Chinese and Ayurvedic medicine, and this led to one of those personal "aha!" moments. Both place great importance on nutrition, and it quickly occurred to me that my high-sugar, low-protein, and very-low-fat diet was making me sick. One thing led to another, and I immersed myself in nutrition research. I learned about the benefits of omega-3 fatty acids, the importance of olive oil, the roles insulin production and inflammation play in disease, and how the right foods could control both. I pumped up my protein intake, cut back on refined carbs, and welcomed nuts, avocados, olive oil, and, yes, even cheese and butter back into my life. I learned to cook, rediscovered the pleasures of food, and found that healthy eating doesn't mean deprivation.

Within a few weeks of changing my diet, I had more energy. I lost weight, and my skin cleared up. Within 2 years, my hair was just as lush as it used to be.

Once I'd healed myself, I wanted to share what I had learned. I trained to become an integrative physician, studying under Andrew Weil, MD, who was among the first to embrace holistic health. Today, I'm the medical director of my own holistic health practice in Atlanta, making food a part of both prevention and cure.

But I'm not the only one who eats this way. As we combed through the tips, recipes, and eating plans from our health professionals, we began to notice a pattern. We found that although personal tastes differ, everyone from the brain doctor to the exercise physiologist follows the same basic eating principles, including these.

Eat a pound of produce a day. It's not difficult. A large apple can easily be a third of a pound. Tomato sauce counts. So do beans and lentils. Studies show that people who have a high intake of fruits and vegetables weigh less and that they are protected against developing diseases such as cancer and heart disease.

Consume lean protein. Your diet should emphasize plant foods but include some dairy, meat, poultry, or fish. Our doctors recommend fish twice a week; plenty of plant-based protein, such as lentils; and small amounts of lean meat, such as grass-fed beef. One Harvard study found that limiting red meat intake to no more than 10.5 ounces per week could prevent 1 in 13 early deaths in women.

Pair your carbs with protein or fat. Carbohydrates are the body's preferred source of energy, but when they're eaten by themselves, they get turned into glucose faster than they would if paired with something that slows digestion, such as a slice of cheese or some oil and vinegar on a salad. Eaten alone, carbohydrates cause a spike in insulin, which is followed by a blood sugar crash that only leaves you hungry for more.

Don't be afraid of fat. Fat is an integral component of every cell in your body. It also helps you absorb fat-soluble nutrients from low-fat foods, keeps skin and hair healthy, and makes your brain work more efficiently. And fat makes food taste good. The key is choosing good fats, such as olive oil. Even the most ardent vegetable lover will agree: A little olive oil, Parmesan cheese, toasted nuts, or even—wait for it—butter on top of steamed asparagus makes the veggie more flavorful.

"Our doctors recommend fish, plant-based protein, and lean meat."

THE EXPERTS' CHOICES

Here are some top tips from physicians. Physicians tend to be a healthier group than most of us. Perhaps it's because they see the result of years of poor eating and not enough exercising. Curious about what doctors actually eat? We were too.

PAMPER YOUR SKIN—FROM WITHIN. "Green and yellow vegetables, such as zucchini and squash or peppers, sautéed in extra virgin olive oil are excellent healthy-skin foods. They help prevent crow's-feet."

—Jessica Wu, MD, assistant clinical professor of dermatology at the University of Southern California Keck School of Medicine

GET HOOKED ON FISH. "A piece of grilled fish—served with a green salad and broccoli tossed with lemon juice, garlic, and olive oil—is a delicious, healthy meal. There's evidence that anti-inflammatory foods like these enhance both physical and emotional health. I choose only sustainable fish, such as sardines, that are low in contaminants."

—Andrew Weil, MD, director of the Arizona Center for Integrative Medicine at the University of Arizona

EXTINGUISH THE FIRE. "Foods low in fat and high in fiber, like oatmeal, beans, and whole grains, help prevent heartburn. Fatty foods, caffeine, alcohol, tomato sauce, peppermint, chocolate, and citrus can trigger it."

—Roshini Raj, MD, gastroenterologist and internist, attending physician at NYU Langone Medical Center

REPLACE RICE. "Buckwheat is not a grain but a fruit seed that's related to rhubarb and sorrel, so it's a suitable replacement for people who are sensitive to wheat, and it's significantly higher in protein than brown rice. Eating buckwheat can lower your risk of developing high cholesterol and high blood pressure. It's rich in flavonoids, which protect against disease. Buckwheat also lowers the risk of diabetes."

—Steven Lamm, MD, internist and faculty member at the New York University School of Medicine

BAKE VEGGIE CHIPS. "Make it a priority to eat colorful foods, even at snack time. My kids and I love to munch on kale chips. They're easy to make: Tear the leaves into bite-size pieces, brush them with olive oil, place them in a single layer on a baking sheet at 300°F, and cook until crisp. Kale contains compounds that can help prevent cancer."

—Lisa Muncy-Pietrzak, MD, internal medicine specialist at the Vitality Center in the Vail Mountain Lodge and Spa in Colorado

TEA UP. "Tea contains an array of flavonoids, potent antioxidant compounds that protect your heart and may guard against infection. I take out my prettiest teacup and brew a pot when I feel like snacking on foods I shouldn't be eating."

—Barbara Quinn, RD, clinical dietitian and diabetes educator at the Community Hospital of the Monterey Peninsula in California

PUMP UP PROTEIN. "It's important for over–30 women to get a concentrated dose of protein at a single meal—at least 20 grams. That's about what you'll find in a 3½-ounce salmon fillet or 2 eggs and 2 slices of whole wheat toast with 1 tablespoon of peanut butter."

—Wayne Westcott, PhD, fitness research director at Quincy College

CHAPTER 18

THE GREENS REVOLUTION

Finally, veggies are no longer an afterthought on Americans' dinner plates, as an explosion of culinary creativity shows how versatile, easy to make, and delicious they can be.

Not so long ago, professional chefs and harried moms alike seemed to lavish most of their culinary efforts on the item at the center of their dinner plates— the inevitable hunk of meat. Vegetables were an afterthought, perfectly adequate for a side dish but rarely the centerpiece and certainly not the most exciting part of the meal. But after years of playing supporting roles, veggies are starting to share the spotlight and, in some venues at least, are even becoming the new divas of dinner.

This quiet revolution can be seen in the growing number of popular veggie-centric cookbooks, restaurants, diet plans, and gorgeous supermarket displays that transform the produce section of many groceries into a garden of delights. (Eataly, a New York City market, even has a "vegetable butcher," who will do the chopping for you on demand.) The reason for this new push is no mystery.

"Research has consistently shown that people who eat larger proportions of fruits and vegetables—particularly vegetables—are healthier," says Marion Nestle, PhD, professor of nutrition, food studies, and public health at New York University.

You don't need to be fully vegetarian or vegan to reap the health benefits. But you do need to consume more vegetables—not spinach pasta or veggie chips, but actual whole vegetables. The key is just to flip the ratio of foods in your diet.

"Instead of an 8-ounce steak and a 4-ounce portion of vegetables, serve 4 ounces of beef and 8 ounces of veggies," advises Michael Pollan in the new edition of his bestseller *Food Rules*. Equally important, eat fewer processed foods while increasing those vegetable servings. As Pollan puts it, "If it came from a plant, eat it. If it was made in a plant, don't."

Restaurants have gotten the message and are amping up their veggie options, and many are finding that it's good for the bottom line. When Andrew Weil, MD (a member of *Prevention*'s editorial advisory board), opened True Food Kitchen in Phoenix in 2008, his restaurant partner and CEO, Sam Fox, was doubtful that the veggie-rich venture would succeed. Now there are three more locations—in Scottsdale, Arizona; Santa Monica, California; and Newport Beach, California—and plans to open four more in San Diego and Denver.

"Sam says he's never seen anything like it," says Dr. Weil. "There are diners who come in four and five times a week. People come up to him on the street and hug him."

Of course, it's one thing to let a chef do all the work and quite another to do your own washing, peeling, and chopping. But with grocery stores stocking more pre-chopped fresh and ready-to-cook frozen veggies, raising your vegetable quotient has never been easier.

The simplest approach, says Mark Bittman, author of *Food Matters* and *How to Cook Everything Vegetarian*, is to change the proportions of ingredients in dishes you cook anyway. "Make frittatas with more vegetables and fewer eggs," he suggests. "Instead of cassoulet that's heavy on meat and light on vegetables, prepare it with lots of beans and veggies and just a little meat for flavor and texture."

VEGGIES IN A SNAP

Does all the prep work keep you from serving vegetables? The following products offer some easy shortcuts.

MANN'S BROCCOLI COLE SLAW: Pile this crunchy medley of shredded broccoli, carrots, and red cabbage on your burger. Or toss it in a light Asian-style vinaigrette to make slaw.

GLORY FOODS KALE GREENS: This prechopped, prewashed kale is picked when it's young and tender. Steam it, toss in a little oil, and add chopped pine nuts. Season to taste.

CASCADIAN FARM PREMIUM BLENDS: Make a 15-minute stir-fry with Chinese-Style Stir-fry Blend (green beans, broccoli, carrots, red peppers, onions, and mushrooms). Toss in a wok with soy sauce and sesame oil.

MELISSA'S STEAMED LENTILS: Normally, lentils take 25 minutes to an hour to cook. These are ready-to-eat. Microwave them in minutes for veggie casseroles—or use cold in a salad.

Or, if you're willing to put in a touch more effort, you can turn your veggies into gourmet fare.

"The range of possibilities is far greater with vegetables than with meat," says Daniel Patterson, chef-owner of the restaurant Coi in San Francisco. "I could give you 500 flavors of plants. You can't get 500 flavors of meat."

NOW GET COOKING! FIVE NEW RECIPES

To discover your own new tastes, try our five outstanding veggie-starring recipes, including an original twist on Surf & Turf that features scallops with a roasted cauliflower "steak." Roasting caramelizes the sugars, bringing out a natural sweetness in the cauliflower, and complements the savory combination of shallots, sun-dried tomatoes, capers, and pine nuts. Drizzle with vinaigrette, and you'll never again ask, "Where's the beef?"—not in this dish, anyway. Bon appetit!

ASPARAGUS AND CHICKEN FRICASSEE

Carrots add sweetness, color, and antioxidants to the polenta, which is made from corn but considered a grain.

Makes 4 servings

¾ pound medium carrots, cut into 1" pieces

1 cup instant polenta

¼ teaspoon salt

¼ teaspoon ground black pepper

2 tablespoons olive oil

1 pound thin-sliced boneless, skinless chicken breasts, cut into 1½" pieces

1 small onion, chopped

8 ounces sliced mushrooms

2 cloves garlic, minced

½ cup dry white wine

1 bunch asparagus, cut into 1½" pieces

1. In a saucepan, cover the carrots with 2" of water. Bring to a boil. Simmer for 15 minutes, until tender. Drain and puree in a food processor until smooth.

2. In the same saucepan, bring 4 cups of water to a boil. Whisk in the polenta. Cook over low heat for 5 minutes, stirring, until thickened. Stir in the carrot puree and season with ⅛ teaspoon salt and ⅛ teaspoon pepper. Keep it warm off the heat.

3. In a large nonstick skillet, heat the oil over medium-high heat. Cook the chicken for 4 minutes in batches, turning, until golden brown and cooked through. Transfer to a plate. Season with ⅛ teaspoon salt and ⅛ teaspoon pepper. Add the onion and cook for 3 minutes, until golden brown. Stir in the mushrooms and cook for 6 minutes, until golden. Add the garlic and cook for 1 minute. Pour in the wine and simmer for 2 minutes, until reduced by half. Stir in the asparagus and cook for 6 minutes, until tender. Return the chicken to the skillet and heat through.

4. Spoon the polenta onto 4 plates and top with the fricassee. Serve immediately.

PER SERVING: 478 calories, 32 g protein, 62 g carbohydrates, 7 g sugars, 10 g total fat, 2 g saturated fat, 6 g fiber, 340 mg sodium

TUSCAN SPINACH DUMPLINGS WITH WHITE BEANS

Spinach stars in these veggie "meatballs." Squeezing out the moisture and rechopping the leaves ensures tenderness.

Makes 6 servings

⅓ cup + ¼ cup all-purpose flour

⅛ teaspoon freshly ground nutmeg

⅛ teaspoon ground black pepper

1 box (10 ounces) frozen chopped spinach, thawed

½ cup part-skim ricotta cheese

½ cup finely grated Parmesan cheese

2 large eggs, beaten

1 can (15 ounces) cannellini beans, rinsed and drained

2 cups reduced-sodium chicken broth

¼ teaspoon red-pepper flakes

1 tablespoon extra virgin olive oil

1 tablespoon fresh lemon juice

1½ ounces sliced prosciutto, torn

1. Bring a large pot of water to a boil.

2. In a small bowl, whisk together ⅓ cup of the flour with the nutmeg and black pepper.

3. In a clean kitchen towel, wrap up the spinach, squeeze out any excess moisture, and finely chop.

4. In a large bowl, stir the spinach, ricotta cheese, Parmesan cheese, eggs, and flour mixture until well combined.

5. In a shallow bowl, put the remaining ¼ cup flour. With wet hands, form the spinach mixture into 30 round dumplings (about 1" diameter and a scant 1 tablespoon each). Roll each dumpling in the flour in batches to coat, shaking off the excess, and arrange on a plate in a single layer.

6. Add the dumplings to the pot and cook at a rolling boil for 5 minutes. With a slotted spoon, transfer to a bowl. Cover and keep warm.

7. In a saucepan, stir together the beans, broth, and red-pepper flakes. Bring to a simmer for 10 minutes, stirring, until heated through.

8. Divide the beans among 6 bowls, and top each with 5 dumplings. Drizzle evenly with the oil and lemon juice. Top with the prosciutto.

PER SERVING: 215 calories, 14 g protein, 19 g carbohydrates, 1 g sugars, 9 g total fat, 4 g sat fat, 4 g fiber, 513 mg sodium

VERY VEGGIE PASTA TOSS

Broccoli slaw blends in with the pasta, making a smaller portion seem ample. One serving satisfies a third of your daily fiber goal.

Makes 6 servings

2 tablespoons olive oil

1 large bell pepper, sliced

1 package (12 ounces) broccoli slaw

2 cups shredded carrots

1 pint cherry tomatoes, halved

3 cloves garlic, minced

½ pound whole wheat angel hair pasta

1–2 tablespoons balsamic vinegar

¼ teaspoon salt

¼ teaspoon black pepper

1. In a large, deep nonstick skillet, heat the oil over medium-high heat. Add the bell pepper, slaw, and carrots and cook for 8 minutes, stirring, until tender. Transfer to a bowl.

2. Add the tomatoes to the skillet and cook for 8 minutes, stirring, until wilted. Add the garlic and cook for 1 minute. Remove the skillet from the heat and set aside.

3. While the vegetables cook, prepare the pasta al dente per the package directions. Reserve ½ cup of the cooking liquid and drain the pasta well.

4. Add the pasta, vegetables, reserved cooking liquid, and vinegar (to taste) to the skillet. Cook over medium-high heat for 5 minutes, stirring, until heated through. Season with the salt and black pepper. Serve immediately.

PER SERVING: 246 calories, 8 g protein, 42 g carbohydrates, 7 g sugars, 6 g total fat, 0.5 g sat fat, 8 g fiber, 150 mg sodium

ROASTED ZUCCHINI NO-NOODLE LASAGNA

Zucchini sliced lengthwise is a perfect swap for noodles, cutting carbs by 39 percent!

Makes 10 servings

2 teaspoons olive oil

1 pound Italian-style poultry sausage, casings removed

6 cups marinara sauce, divided

2½ pounds large zucchini, trimmed and sliced lengthwise into ¼" to ½" slices

1 pound frozen peas, thawed

3 large eggs

1 cup chopped parsley

1 cup part-skim ricotta cheese

⅓ cup finely grated Parmesan cheese

¼ teaspoon salt

¼ teaspoon ground black pepper

1. In a large nonstick skillet, heat the oil over medium-high heat. Add the sausage and cook for 6 minutes, until no longer pink. Stir in 4 cups of the marinara and simmer for 10 minutes, until thickened.

2. Preheat the broiler. Line 2 large sheet pans with nonstick foil and coat with cooking spray. Working in batches, arrange the zucchini slices in a single layer on the prepared pans and coat the tops with cooking spray. Broil 6" from the heat for 5 minutes, until golden. Flip the zucchini and broil for 3 minutes, until golden. Transfer to a plate.

3. In a food processor, pulse to combine the peas, eggs, parsley, ricotta cheese, and Parmesan cheese. Season with the salt and pepper.

4. Preheat the oven to 350°F and coat a 13" x 9" baking pan with cooking spray.

5. In the bottom of the pan, spoon one-quarter of the meat sauce and top with one-quarter of the zucchini. Spread one-third of the pea mixture evenly on top. Repeat layering in same manner 2 more times. Finish with an additional layer of sauce and zucchini. Cover the pan with foil and bake for 25 minutes. Remove the cover and bake for 10 minutes, until the top is golden and firm to the touch. Let it stand for 20 minutes before serving. Warm the remaining 2 cups marinara and serve with the lasagna.

PER SERVING: 258 calories, 21 g protein, 25 g carbohydrates, 11 g sugar, 9 g total fat, 3 g saturated fat, 6 g fiber, 918 mg sodium

SEA SCALLOP SURF & TURF

Cauliflower can be your low-cal "turf" in a Surf & Turf meal. Once roasted, it has a meaty texture that contrasts nicely with delicate scallops.

Makes 4 servings

1 head cauliflower (about 2 pounds), stem removed

¼ teaspoon + ⅛ teaspoon salt

¼ teaspoon + ⅛ teaspoon ground black pepper

12 sea scallops (about 1 pound), side muscle removed

2 tablespoons olive oil

2 shallots, finely chopped

2 tablespoons capers, rinsed and drained

1 tablespoon chopped dry-packed sun-dried tomatoes

2 tablespoons sherry wine vinegar or fresh lemon juice

¼ cup chopped parsley

2 tablespoons pine nuts, toasted

1. Preheat the oven to 425°F. Line a sheet pan with nonstick foil and coat lightly with cooking spray.

2. Slice the head of cauliflower crosswise to create flat disks (½" thick) and arrange on the prepared pan. Coat the tops with cooking spray and season with ¼ teaspoon each of the salt and pepper. Roast in the upper third of the oven for 25 minutes, turning once with a spatula, until golden brown on both sides and tender. Turn off the heat, leaving the pan in the oven to keep warm.

3. Pat the scallops dry and season with ⅛ teaspoon each of the salt and pepper. In a large nonstick skillet, heat the oil over medium-high heat. When the oil is hot, add the scallops and cook for 4 minutes, turning once, until golden brown on both sides and cooked through. Transfer to a plate.

4. Add the shallots, capers, and sun-dried tomatoes to the skillet, and cook for 2 minutes, stirring, over medium heat, until the shallots are tender. Stir in the vinegar. Return the scallops to the pan, sprinkle with the parsley, and heat through for 2 minutes.

5. On 4 plates, arrange the cauliflower and top with the scallops. Spoon the juices from the skillet over the scallops and sprinkle with the nuts.

PER SERVING: 232 calories, 22 g protein, 12 g carbohydrates, 6 g sugars, 11 g total fat, 2 g saturated fat, 2 g fiber, 578 mg sodium

VEGGIE IMPOSTORS

Not every product that boasts "spinach" on the label is even remotely like a serving of the real thing. Basic rule: If it doesn't look like a vegetable, it probably isn't.

SUN-DRIED TOMATO WRAPS: The tomatoes provide little more than coloring. And watch out for sodium levels, which can soar. "If you want vegetables, stuff your wrap with them, but don't expect to get them in the wrap itself," says Karen Ansel, RD.

PIZZA: No joke: In 2011, Congress ruled that pizza counts as a veggie in school lunches, because a slice has about 2 tablespoons of tomato paste. But with all that crust and cheese (refined carbs and saturated fats), most pizza is not ideal.

VEGGIE CHIPS: Don't be misled by photos on the bag. Check to see if real veggies are near the top of the ingredients list. They probably aren't. And because they're dehydrated and not as filling as the real thing, you eat more calories.

SPINACH PASTA: Manufacturers hope that spinach's health halo will lead you to buy their pasta. But read labels carefully before you do. Put a product back if the Nutrition Facts panel doesn't boast 25 percent of your vitamin A and 2 grams of fiber.

"I could give you 500 flavors of plants.
You can't get 500 flavors of meat."

—Daniel Patterson, chef-owner of the restaurant Coi in San Francisco

CHAPTER 19

A NEW CULTURE

There are 100 trillion good bacteria in your gut, working wonders to help keep you healthy. Here's how probiotics and prebiotics work and what you need to know.

Probiotics are the latest craze in the food industry, turning up in everything from pizza to chocolate. They now tally $20 billion in global sales, expanding at 20 to 30 percent a year. If you're not already consuming them in some form, chances are you will be soon.

"Probiotics are the new vitamins," says Shekhar Challa, MD, a gastroenterologist in Topeka, Kansas, and the author of *Probiotics for Dummies.*

That's a bold statement, because probiotics are actually living microbes—specifically, beneficial bacteria that promote human health if consumed in large enough quantities. For germophobic Americans, it's a revolutionary concept. But the 100 trillion microbes that live in your large intestine do dozens of good things for you. They process indigestible fibers and help keep bowel function regular. They produce a number of vitamins, including B_6, B_{12}, and K_2, and aid in the absorption of minerals such as iron, calcium, and magnesium. Equally important, they help fend off bad bacteria such as salmonella and

The microbes that turn milk into yogurt and kefir are the most beneficial, and they seem to thrive in dairy.

E. coli, which can cause diarrhea and, in extreme cases, severe anemia, kidney failure, and death.

"The intestines are a war zone, where beneficial and harmful bacteria are fighting to establish predominance," says Venket Rao, PhD, emeritus professor of nutritional sciences at the University of Toronto. The key is for the good guys to outnumber the bad. If you want to give them a competitive edge, a regular supply of probiotics can help.

The payoff can extend well beyond your gut, and your immune system is a prime beneficiary. In a Swedish study of 262 workers, those who took probiotics for 80 days were 42 percent less likely to take a sick day for an upper respiratory infection or gastrointestinal disease. Regular doses can help reduce vaginal and urinary tract infections. If you're prone to allergies or eczema, probiotics might even help tamp down an overactive immune system. They accomplish all this by producing their own form of antibiotics, blocking pathogens from adhering to the gut, and spurring production of chemical messengers called cytokines, which communicate with the immune system throughout the body. Probiotics might even enhance your mood, thanks to a similar cross talk with the central nervous system.

So the conclusion is simple, right? Take probiotics. Unfortunately, it's not that easy. There are more than 3,000 species of good bacteria in your gut, and each has its own talents. The challenge is that cultures you're consuming might not be the ones that reduce colds or fight diarrhea. And they have to be handled correctly, so they aren't killed during processing or storage.

"No more than 10 percent of products that claim to be probiotic have been proven in human trials," says Gregor Reid, PhD, chairman of human microbiology and probiotics at the Lawson Health Research Institute.

So what's a shopper to do?

BE CULTURED

The microbes that turn milk into yogurt and kefir are among the most beneficial, and they seem to thrive in dairy.

"Milk contains compounds called oligosaccha-rides [complex carbohydrates] that the bacteria feed on," says Roger A. Clemens, DrPH, adjunct professor at the University of Southern California. Dairy products are also kept chilled, which is important for heat-sensitive organisms, and are only weakly acidic, another plus. (Bacteria can perish in the strongly acidic environment of the stomach, but dairy provides protection.) Just make sure the container says "live and active cultures." Dead bacteria won't help. The more reliable brands tell you which specific bacteria they contain.

While the strains in most yogurt brands are beneficial, Dannon's Activia yogurt and DanActive drink are among the rare products backed by published, peer-reviewed studies. Kefir contains even more strains than yogurt.

BEYOND THE DINNER TABLE

Probiotics aren't just in food anymore. They're turning up in breath mints, mouthwash, hand sanitizer, and cleaning products. Why? If you want to control bad bacteria in your gut, you might also want to keep them in check in your mouth, on your hands, and on kitchen counters.

But do these products work? We won't vouch for them all. But in an informal test at *Prevention*'s offices (using a device to measure the biofilm that harbors bad bacteria), the PIP line of probiotic cleaning products outperformed conventional cleaners on a microwave keypad, a computer keyboard, a bathroom floor, and even an employee's hands.

Try PIP's Pure Clean Hand Gel. It combines alcohol with beneficial bacteria to keep the bad germs at bay longer. ($7.95 for 2 ounces; pipcleaners.com)

LEARN TO PICKLE

Microbes are responsible for fermentation, turning cabbage into sauerkraut, cucumbers into sour pickles, and soybeans into miso. For thousands of years, fermented foods have been staples of the human diet. But we eat far fewer of these foods today, and when we do, modern processing often kills off the good bacteria.

"Stores can't have jars exploding on shelves when bacteria produce gas, so manufacturers pasteurize sauerkraut and pickles," says Mary Ellen Sanders, PhD, executive director of the International Scientific Association for Probiotics and Prebiotics. "Unless you're pulling your pickles out of a crock in a deli or buying them from a small local producer who labels them 'raw fermented,' you're not getting live microbes."

Make your own, says Sandor Ellix Katz, author of *The Art of Fermentation*. For sauerkraut, slice cabbage thin, massage it in a bowl with 1 tablespoon of salt to draw out the water, and store it in the brine you've just created. Wait a week or more while it ferments. It's really that simple! Just be sure to keep the kraut completely covered in the brine to prevent rotting caused by bad bacteria. Robyn Jasko, the author of *Homesweet Homegrown*, recommends a type of jar called Pickl-It (pickl-it.com), which has an airlock that helps to keep bad bacteria out and good bacteria in.

AVOID MARKETING HYPE

Probiotics are now being added to lots of unfermented foods too, including cookies, pizza crust, coffee beans, and powdered smoothie mixes. But unless the label promises "live and active cultures," don't count on them—particularly in products that require heating, such as coffee and pizza. High temperatures are likely to destroy the bacteria.

Chocolate is one product in which added probiotics do well. Attune Foods makes three varieties with beneficial levels of tested strains. Find them in the dairy case at chains such as Safeway.

H ere's another great use for probiotics. A full **30 percent of people get diarrhea when taking antibiotics.** If you're one (or if you don't know and don't care to find out), probiotics might help.

A recent study in the *Journal of the American Medical Association* suggests that you can reduce your risk of the unpleasant side effect by **42 percent** by eating foods with active cultures of these "friendly" bacteria. Take kefir (try Lifeway's frozen or regular) with your next antibiotic.

GIVE YOURSELF A BOOST

Throughout most of human history, getting enough good bacteria was no problem. But today we live in a sanitized world. If you need extra help—for example, if you have chronic constipation (63 million Americans do) or you're taking antibiotics, which kill good and bad bacteria alike—probiotic supplements can provide steady, reliable relief. Earlier this year, a study in the *Journal of the American Medical Association* concluded that patients on antibiotics can reduce the associated risk of diarrhea by 42 percent if they take probiotics at the same time.

Proven brands include Culturelle (for diarrhea) and Align (for inflammatory bowel syndrome). See "Pick Your Pills Wisely" on page 214 for advice on picking a supplement that will help you.

EAT PREBIOTICS

For colonies to thrive, you need to create favorable living conditions for them. One of the best ways to do that is to consume a diet rich in fruits and vegetables.

"Processed foods contain preservatives, which are antimicrobial by definition," Dr. Reid says. By contrast, many natural whole foods include prebiotics, or foods that the good microbes themselves feed on—namely, insoluble fibers that people cannot digest but bacteria can. These fibers are in a variety of foods, including onions, bananas, asparagus, leeks, garlic, artichokes, wheat, oats, and soybeans.

Prebiotics are being added to some packaged foods too. Look for terms such as inulin, FOS, GOS, or polydextrose on the ingredient list.

LACE UP YOUR GYM SHOES

There are so many reasons to exercise—to reduce your blood pressure, build strong bones, and boost mood, to name just a few. But whoever mentions keeping your gut bacteria healthy?

"These organisms replicate about every 20 minutes," Dr. Clemens says. Exercise stimulates gut motility, which benefits good bacteria by regularly

PICK YOUR PILLS WISELY

Not all supplements are equally effective. Here are some things to look for on the label. (Check with your doctor first to make sure a particular product will help your condition.)

CFUS: This means "colony forming units," and there should be at least a billion.

STRAINS: Seek out specific bacteria that will help your problem. For general health, take a brand that contains both a Lactobacillus and a Bifidobacterium.

GUARANTEE OF ACTIVITY: This should include an expiration date, plus directions on how to handle the product at home. Some probiotics are stable at room temperature, but all benefit from cooler temps.

ACID RESISTANCE: Certain strains can be stabilized to survive stomach acids. Others cannot. The bottle should say "acid stabilized" or "microencapsulated."

PREBIOTICS: Some brands include ready-made food sources for the bacteria.

removing toxins that might harm them. By the way, bowel movements are also a general indicator of how healthy these colonies are. "If you're getting adequate fiber and are physically active, you should have more frequent bowel movements that are larger, softer, and lighter in color," says Dr. Clemens.

Here's a surprising fact: Half the volume of your bowel movements is not food waste but bacteria. You have several pounds of these microbes in your gut at any time.

Thirty to 60 minutes of exercise a day will usually do the trick, says Dr. Clemens. "It's another reason to get out and walk."

CHAPTER 20

FOODS THAT FIGHT PAIN

Science is starting to recognize that foods can relieve pain as well as—or even better than—drugs.

Chronic pain affects 116 million American adults. That's more than a third of the US population. And while pain pills reduce suffering, they can be addictive and produce side effects. Worse, they often fail to eliminate the true cause of the pain.

"No matter how well you prescribe medication, chronic sufferers don't get complete relief," says James N. Dillard, MD, author of *The Chronic Pain Solution*. "It's an enormous problem, and the medical community is doing a bad job solving it."

But there is an alternative, and it's right in your kitchen. Certain foods ease aches by fighting inflammation, blocking pain signals, and even healing underlying disease.

"Almost always, if we find pharmaceuticals doing the trick, we'll find a plant doing the same trick—and doing it more safely," says botanist James A. Duke,

PhD, author of *The Green Pharmacy Guide to Healing Foods*.

But before you can reap these rewards, you have to quit the junk food that riles up your body's pain system. The typical Western-style diet is heavy on foods that promote inflammation, including highly processed foods and refined carbs. No fruit, vegetable, or herb by itself can alleviate your pain if you don't change the pattern of your diet to reduce processed food and increase whole foods. This might not be easy, says Peter Abaci, MD, medical director of the Bay Area Pain and Wellness Center in Los Gatos, California. "But if you stay committed to a good nutrition plan, you might be able to say good-bye to pain."

THE Rx: CHERRIES

The target: arthritis and muscle pain
The dose: 45 daily

Compounds in cherries called anthocyanins—the same phytonutrients that give cherries their rich ruby hue—are powerful antioxidants that work in two ways to tamp down pain.

"They block inflammation, and they inhibit pain enzymes, just like aspirin, naproxen, and other nonsteroidal anti-inflammatories," says Muraleedharan Nair, PhD, natural products chemist at Michigan State University's College of Agricultural and Natural Resources.

One study in the *Journal of Nutrition* showed that people who ate a bowl of cherries for breakfast reduced a major marker of inflammation by 25 percent. Other researchers found less muscle pain in runners who drank 12 ounces of tart cherry juice twice daily for 7 days before a distance run.

THE Rx: EDAMAME

The target: arthritis
The dose: ¼ cup daily

When it comes to culinary fixes for pain, osteoarthritis poses a challenge. Wear and tear on the joints—the kind that leaves cartilage tattered and bones grinding against one another—is not reversible. Still, there's hope for relief.

Researchers from Oklahoma State University gave participants either 40 grams of soy protein (about ¼ cup of shelled edamame) or milk-based protein for 3 months. At the study's end, pain was reduced for those who ate soy protein but not for those in the milk protein group.

"I'm talking about tofu, tempeh, other fermented forms of whole soy—not soy protein isolates, which you commonly see in processed snacks," says Dr. Dillard. Cooking with tofu is simple as long as you know the basics. Silken tofu is soft and often used in creamy dressings, soups, and desserts; firm tofu is typically cooked like meat—say, marinated and grilled.

THE Rx: GINGER

The target: migraines, arthritis and sore muscles
The dose: ¼ teaspoon daily

This spicy root is a traditional stomach soother, easing seasickness and nausea. It's believed to work by breaking up intestinal gas and possibly blocking a receptor in the gut that induces vomiting. But there are good reasons to eat ginger even when you're not doubled over. Another natural aspirin impersonator and anti-inflammatory, it can offer relief from migraines, arthritis pain, and muscle aches.

There are plenty of ways to include ginger in your diet. Add it grated into Asian dishes, smoothies, and juice. Or make ginger tea by placing sliced, peeled gingerroot in boiling water and letting it steep for 15 minutes. For ginger lemonade, combine grated gingerroot, lemon juice, and honey with ice water.

THE Rx: CRANBERRY JUICE

The target: ulcers
The dose: 1 cup daily

Ulcers are the result of a pathogen called *H. pylori*, which attacks the protective lining of the stomach or small intestine. Antibiotics are the usual cure, but you can help prevent ulcers in the first place by drinking cranberry juice, thanks to its ability to block *H. pylori* from adhering to the stomach lining. One study found that just under a cup a day for 3 weeks eliminated almost 20 percent of all cases of *H. pylori* infection—without drugs. But the juice becomes inflammatory when it's loaded with sugar, so grab a bottle of 100 percent natural cranberry juice. If it's too bitter, add water or a natural sweetener such as stevia.

THE Rx: SALMON, HERRING, AND SARDINES

The target: achy back, neck, and joints

The dose: two or three 3-ounce servings weekly

Eating fish low in mercury and high in omega-3 fatty acids can help relieve back pain. Here's why: In a healthy back, blood vessels at the edge of spinal disks transport crucial nutrients to those disks. If blood flow is diminished, the disks lose their source of oxygen and other nutrients, and they begin to degenerate, says Neal D. Barnard, MD, author of *Foods That Fight Pain*. Omega-3s help by improving blood flow and tamping down inflammation in blood vessels and nerves.

But for the full effect, you might need supplements. One study in the journal *Surgical Neurology* found that taking 1,200 milligrams or more of EPA and DHA per day could reduce both back and neck pain. And there are added bonuses: "Any amount of fish oil is beneficial for cardiovascular protection and mood elevation," says Joseph C. Maroon, MD, the study's lead researcher. A study in the journal *Pain* found that people are more aware of their discomfort when they're glum.

THE Rx: HOT PEPPERS

The target: arthritis

The dose: $\frac{1}{2}$ teaspoon of powder daily

The same peppers that singe your tongue and bring tears to your eyes can take away pain. An ingredient in hot peppers called capsaicin does the trick by stimulating nerve endings and depleting a chemical that relays pain signals. You can buy capsaicin-containing creams at most pharmacies, says Dr. Duke,

A NATURAL CURE FOR PAIN

New research shows that an ancient therapy can significantly decrease pain. Cupping, which is a close cousin of acupuncture, involves placing glass cups on your body (on either the affected area or the acupuncture points used to treat it) to create suction. While it might sound odd, cupping reduced chronic neck pain by an average of 45 percent among people in a 2011 study from the University of Duisburg-Essen in Germany. Here are the details.

WHY IT WORKS: The suction caused by cupping is meant to free up and balance the flow of qi (pronounced CHEE), or life energy, in the body, says Bryn Clark, a licensed acupuncturist and diplomate of Oriental medicine. It also seems to improve blood circulation.

HOW IT'S DONE: The practitioner might create suction either by using a flame to burn the oxygen from the cup and then applying the cup to your skin or by placing the cup on you first and then removing the air through a valve. Any bruises that result clear up within 5 to 10 days.

WHO CAN BENEFIT: Practitioners have traditionally treated many ailments with cupping therapy. Clark uses it—often along with acupuncture—to treat pain, colds and sinus problems, high blood pressure, asthma, hot flashes, arthritis, painful or irregular periods, and more.

Find a practitioner by searching the National Certification Commission for Acupuncture and Oriental Medicine's directory at nccaom.org.

who uses capsaicin to alleviate his own arthritis pain.

Though topical relief is most effective for arthritis, eating hot peppers also yields pain-fighting benefits. Dr. Duke adds peppers to soups and sprinkles chili sauce on his food. The hotter the pepper, the more capsaicin it contains. But after handling hot peppers, wash your hands thoroughly. A towel wet with milk cuts the pepper better than water. If you touch your face before that, you'll understand why capsaicin is the main ingredient in Mace.

THE Rx: TURMERIC

The target: achy joints and colitis (inflammation of the colon)

The dose: 1 tablespoon daily

This essential curry spice has been used for years in Ayurvedic medicine to relieve pain and speed up digestion. But researchers like it for another reason: its anti-inflammatory properties, courtesy of a substance called curcumin.

"Turmeric can protect the body from tissue destruction and joint inflammation and also preserve good nerve cell function," Dr. Abaci says.

Not a fan of curry? Sprinkle turmeric on salad dressings, soups, cooked grains, and vegetables. Or get an even heftier dose by taking a turmeric supplement. (Make sure the label says it contains 95 percent curcuminoids.) And note: When you cook with turmeric, use the pepper mill.

"Turmeric and black pepper should always go together," Dr. Dillard says. "The piperine in black pepper releases curcumin from the spice."

THE Rx: YOGURT

The target: IBS

The dose: one or two 8-ounce containers daily

For the roughly 20 percent of Americans who have irritable bowel syndrome, stomach pain is a given. But help might come in the form of a bug—billions of bugs, actually. Several bacterial strains that are often in yogurt (especially *B. infantis* and *L. acidophilus*) reduce pain, inflammation, and bloating, according to a 2010 review. Another study found similar results with *B. lactis*.

But shop smart. Not every yogurt contains probiotics. Look for a brand with "live and active cultures." Vegans can get their daily dose from probiotic-enriched soy yogurt.

THE Rx: MINT

The target: IBS and headaches

The dose: 1 cup of tea daily

Chewing on peppermint can freshen your breath, but there's another reason you should try the herb. The menthol in peppermint helps prevent muscle spasms, one of the reasons peppermint oil effectively treats irritable bowel syndrome. The oil is also useful for relieving headaches. Rub some on your temples or wrists and breathe in the minty scent.

Dr. Duke recommends brewing mint tea for any type of pain. Pour boiling water over peppermint leaves and steep until the tea is as strong as you like. Add wintergreen leaves for an extra pain-fighting boost. A compound in wintergreen called methyl salicylate blocks the enzymes that cause inflammation and pain.

"You could call it herbal aspirin," he says. A final squeeze of lemon will help you extract as many pain-reducing chemicals as possible from the plants.

THE Rx: COFFEE

The target: headaches

The dose: two 4-ounce cups

Coffee isn't just a morning pick-me-up. It's good medicine.

"Caffeine helps reduce pain by narrowing the dilated blood vessels that develop with headaches," says Andrew Weil, MD, founder and director of the Arizona Center for Integrative Medicine. And coffee delivers a one-two punch by reducing pain-promoting compounds and amplifying the effect of other pain relievers too. But be warned: If you're a java junkie, too much caffeine can have the opposite effect. When you quit, you can get withdrawal headaches. Coffee works as a headache reliever only if you don't consume it regularly.

CHAPTER 21

SPLENDOR
IN THE GLASS

Having a few drinks made writer Judith Newman feel upbeat and in control, an escape from the stressed-out, irritable person she was without a cocktail in hand. But then she began to worry that her happy habit was something she couldn't live without. In her own words...

I am running on the treadmill and sobbing. Have you ever noticed how songs are more meaningful when the blood flow to your brain is amped up? Today, it's Neil Diamond who's hitting me hard, as I listen to him croon: Red, red wine, go to my head, make me forget that I still need her so...

I've had a lot of worries this past year. Husband-health concerns. Kid concerns. My father dying a year ago, and not long thereafter, my mother, whom I loved very much—and I still need her so.

But the red, red wine—or in my case, the vodka—has been helping me forget, a little too much and too often. I'm a nice girl from a teeto-taling family, but, as life's pressures have mounted, I've begun feeling as though I've gone from enjoying one Cosmo (or two or three) at the end of the day to *needing* one.

But is it really so bad to enjoy a glass of something in the evening? Last year, after all, the Centers for Disease Control and Prevention declared moderate drinking one of four lifestyle behaviors that help people live longer. The other three: eating a healthy diet, exercising, and not smoking.

The CDC (along with the USDA and the National Institutes of Health) defines "moderate drinking" as no more than one drink per day for most women, up to two for most men. One drink is defined as 5 ounces of wine or 1.5 fluid ounces of distilled spirits, which to me sounds not so much like "drinking" as "licking the glass." A classic vodka gimlet, for instance, calls for 1.5 to 2 ounces of vodka, but try making one and see if you don't end up pouring twice that amount.

But wait a second: I'm a pretty big girl—5-foot-8, a size 10. Does this mean that compared with a man my size and weight, I'm a big drunk, and he's just a bon vivant?

Very handily, I happen upon a checklist endorsed by Harvard called the CAGE test, designed to identify problem drinkers. The questions are:

1. Have you ever felt you should <u>C</u>ut down on your drinking?

2. Have people <u>A</u>nnoyed you by criticizing your drinking?

3. Have you ever felt <u>G</u>uilty or bad about your drinking?

4. Have you ever had a drink first thing in the morning to steady your nerves, get rid of a hangover, or as an <u>E</u>ye-opener?

"If you responded 'yes' to any one of these questions, you may have a drinking problem," the questionnaire reads. "If you responded 'yes' to more than one question, it's highly likely that a problem exists."

It is that fourth one that has me at the tipping point. A celebratory gin and tonic before noon with friends that might, coincidentally, counteract a hang-over. Does that qualify?

I take some comfort in the fact that I am not alone. While the National

A little bit of alcohol can go a long way for good health, but moderation is key. Enjoying a serving of alcohol (5 ounces of wine, 12 ounces of beer, or 1.5 ounces of hard liquor) will help you with the following.

STRENGTHEN YOUR HEART. One drink a day can help reduce your risk of heart disease by 25 percent, thanks to its raising "good" HDL cholesterol.

STAY MENTALLY SHARP. Moderate drinkers are 23 percent less likely to develop dementia, Alzheimer's disease, and other forms of cognitive impairment.

STAVE OFF STROKE. Women who have no more than one drink a day are less susceptible to having a stroke.

AVOID GALLSTONES. Research shows that sipping a daily serving of alcohol reduces the risk of gallstones in women by 20 percent.

KEEP DIABETES AT BAY. Some studies suggest that small amounts of alcohol can have beneficial effects on insulin and triglyceride concentrations.

Institute on Alcohol Abuse and Alcoholism has long stated that a woman's drinking life peaks in her twenties and thirties, several studies suggest that drinking among women in their forties and fifties has been underreported. While there has been a decrease in binge drinking in this middle-age group since 2000, there has been an increase in hidden forms of drinking, such as tippling alone at home. And yes, guilty as charged. That's when I decide I need a few more answers.

WHAT'S UP, DOC?

My first move is to schedule a meeting with Denise Szczucki, MD, a psychiatrist specializing in addictions, at New York City's Caron drug and alcohol treatment center. While national statistics show that there are more male alcoholics, at a ratio of about five to two, Dr. Szczucki doubts their accuracy.

"I think female alcoholism is underreported, because, well, women don't come to the attention of the law in the way men do," she says. "They're not getting into bar fights. They're drinking at home, quietly."

I used to drink only when I was out with friends. Now I'm reaching for the bottle the moment my twin boys come home from school. I reason that nobody could listen to a 10-year-old explicate Pokémon and its powers stone-cold sober. Drink number two is poured around the time my husband reminds me of the litany of tasks I've failed to accomplish domestically that day. And in the past few weeks, drinks three and four have come about when I reach for the phone to joke about it with my mother—and she isn't there.

Dr. Szczucki gives me a thorough medical and psychological examination and orders a blood test with two screens for alcoholism. The mean corpuscular volume (MCV) is a measure of the size of red blood cells. Red blood cells are unusually large with B vitamin deficiencies. These deficiencies—particularly a lack of B_7, B_{12}, and folate—are signs of alcohol abuse, because alcohol interferes with their absorption. Then she orders liver-enzyme screening tests. SGOT, SGPT, and GGT are intrinsic enzymes in the liver, but when people drink too much, these enzymes leak into the blood. High blood levels of these enzymes are associated with liver damage.

She also looks at me funny. Later on, I discover she's scrutinizing me for overt signs of too much drinking: flushing, sweating, shaky hands and rosacea. (Excessive drinking doesn't give you this skin inflammation, but if you already have rosacea, drinking can cause it to flare up.)

At the end of the appointment, Dr. Szczucki asks me to record my alcohol consumption over the course of a week. She shows me how to use a Breathalyzer, which entails breathing into the machine 20 minutes after I drink. Breathalyzers measure blood alcohol concentration, or BAC. Alcohol is absorbed into the bloodstream via the stomach and the small intestine; it then moves across the membranes of the lungs' air sacs. It does not change its chemical composition. That's why the alcohol concentration in one's breath is directly related to its concentration in the blood. Therefore, a reading of 0.04 percent on the Breathalyzer means that 0.04 percent of my blood is alcohol.

"I can stop drinking for a month relatively easily, right? Right?"

She also instructs me to monitor my blood pressure and heart rate with a blood-pressure cuff. When we drink a little bit, our blood pressure rises, and our dilated blood vessels fill up more fully with higher pressures. That's why our faces flush (blood rises to the surface), and we become more voluble and "sparkly."

Like every closet hypochondriac, I rather enjoy my new gadgets, though it's somewhat of a problem explaining to my children what I'm doing. So I don't. "Mommy, are you sick?" Gus asks as he sees me anxiously huffing into the Breathalyzer. "No," I want to say, "I have to do this because lately Mommy's been a little too cheerful."

7 DAYS LATER

After a week of Breathalyzing, I return to Dr. Szczucki, and the results both surprise and calm me. My heart rate remained about the same as it is when I'm not drinking, and my blood pressure was unaffected too. It was slightly elevated on the occasion when I'd had three glasses of white wine without anything to eat all day, but barely: 140/90, compared with 130/80, my usual.

The Breathalyzer scores went like this: 0.04 percent, 0.01 percent, 0.04 percent, 0.03 percent, 0.02 percent, and 0.04 percent, which means I didn't even approach the legal limit in New York State, which is 0.08 percent.

"A 0.04 percent is consistent with two or three drinks, the point where you're a little euphoric and talkative. It's the fun point," Dr. Szczucki says rather cheerfully.

So why do I feel as though I'm getting more headachy and queasy when I drink? In addition to the differences in the ways women and men metabolize alcohol (see "A Woman's Body on Alcohol" on page 232), there's the inevitable march of time. Tolerance for alcohol decreases with age. I'm in my fifties, and while I wasn't a big drinker at 25 by any means, I could drink more then than I do now, with less insomnia and fewer headaches as a result. That's partly because the aging brain becomes more sensitive to all drugs, including alcohol, although it's not clear why.

At this point, Dr. Szczucki and I agree that I will abstain entirely from alcohol for a full month, so I can see what it feels like.

"You might find it hard to go to sleep," she says. That's not unusual, because even when people aren't addicted by conventional standards, the brain and nervous system need time to revert to the state they were in before the drinking began. "And I tell my patients to expect alcohol cravings and plan for them: Call a friend, go for a walk," she adds. "Have alternative rewards in place."

MY 30-DAY TEST

When I get home, I feel quite relieved. Now that I know I'm not physically addicted, I can do a month relatively easily, right? Right?

There are 2 days of no liquor. Then...

THE DOWNSIDE OF BOTTOMS UP

To determine if you're becoming physically addicted to alcohol, examine the four classic symptoms below. Do they describe you?

CRAVING: A strong need or urge to drink

PHYSICAL DEPENDENCE: Withdrawal symptoms, such as nausea, sweating, shakiness, and anxiety, after stopping drinking

LOSS OF CONTROL: Not being able to stop drinking once drinking has begun

TOLERANCE: The need to drink greater amounts of alcohol to get "high"

If one or more of these descriptions fit your experience, speak with your family physician for a definitive diagnosis. Should the two of you determine that treatment is needed, available options include inpatient and outpatient facilities, medication, and counseling, used singly or in combination.

Reputable independent organizations to consider contacting for counseling and referrals include the following.

Alcoholics Anonymous: AA.org

National Drug and Alcohol Treatment Referral Routing Service: 800-662-HELP (4357)

Substance Abuse and Mental Health Services Administration: samhsa.gov

Aunt Alberta's 85th birthday. I am uninvited to the party because my aunt's daughter isn't talking to me. Family angst; feel sorry for myself. Drink.

Visit a friend in a Boston hospital who's getting a bone marrow transplant. Is a life-or-death transplant the time to quit drinking? No. Drink.

Day after transplant. Everything went well. Have to toast. Drink.

Two days with nothing to drink! Nothing!

Friends from England come to visit. Is it possible not to drink around British people? No. Drink.

Take family to see *The Lion King.* By intermission, both sons have their hands over their ears and are whining that it's too loud. We leave. I should have never had them. Drink.

Sleepover party with nine 10-year-old boys, three with ADHD, in my cramped New York City apartment. About the time one of them is spitting blood into my sink (after somehow splitting his lip open while sandwiched between two mattresses by his buddies and repeatedly jumped on), I leave them to reenact *Lord of the Flies* while I break out the bourbon.

Finally, I steel myself and get some resolve. I wait until my husband is away on a 2-week trip, because "no husband" equals "much less stress," and put all the bottles of liquor in storage. I also decide, as Dr. Szczucki advised, to give myself little treats along the way.

The first treat is a bunch of new beauty products. This is great, until I realize that this new facial scrub smells so deliciously like a piña colada that I want to run out of the shower and grab a coconut and a straw. Fine. So I graduate from the scrub to really good dark chocolate—thus ensuring that any weight loss I might experience from the saved booze calories will be negated by my accelerated Godiva habit.

That's when I decide that my real reward should be a few new trinkets. I limit myself to sales online. So much great stuff, so cheap!

In 3 days, I spend $3,000.

Do I really need a professional clothing steamer that barely fits in my closet?

Well, apparently I do, what with the closetful of new clothes.

"Your experience is typical," says Dr. Szczucki after I slink back to her office.

"Even though any physical withdrawal is over after a week, sometimes people substitute one less-than-desirable behavior for another. So you need to avoid the situations that trigger cravings."

Which in my case would pretty much mean moving out of my house, because the biggest trigger is my family.

MY NEW, DRY(ER) LIFE

In the end, I was entirely booze-free for only 2 consecutive weeks. But even within that short amount of time, here's what happened: My headaches disappeared. I didn't have to pee every hour, which ensured a more restful sleep. My moods were more stable; I did not ping-pong back and forth between Falsely Jolly Mommy and Homicidal Mommy. I did not lose any weight—that damned chocolate—but I didn't gain any either, and because I wasn't lagging in the morning, I could exercise more.

I also had the same blood tests taken to see if there was any difference in my MCV or liver-enzyme tests. There wasn't, which would again prove that I never had much of a problem in the first place, right? Not so fast, says Dr. Szczucki.

"Even with normal blood work, an alcohol dependency can develop if you

A WOMAN'S BODY ON ALCOHOL

Women are more vulnerable to alcohol's effects than men are, ounce for ounce.

Women have about 50 percent less alcohol dehydrogenase, which is the enzyme that metabolizes alcohol in the stomach, than men do. This means that women absorb 100 percent of what they drink.

Women also have less water and more fat in their bodies, so alcohol is more concentrated in the female bloodstream.

LIQUID CALORIES

Just because something is served in a glass doesn't mean it doesn't contain plenty of calories.

BLOODY MARY: **1.5 ounces vodka: 120 calories**

COSMO: **1.5 ounces vodka, 0.75 ounces triple sec: 200 calories**

MARGARITA: **1.4 ounces tequila, 0.7 ounces Cointreau: 155 calories**

MARTINI: **1.5 ounces gin, 0.5 ounces dry vermouth: 119 calories**

RED WINE: **5 ounces: 125 calories**

WHITE WINE: **5 ounces: 121 calories**

meet the clinical criteria, which is that you have a loss of control over the amount you're drinking and develop a greater tolerance to alcohol, because you're drinking more. You did exhibit signs of mild alcohol withdrawal, which is also a sign of dependence. Even if you're not physically addicted, you can still be psychologically dependent, which means that you crave alcohol, feel you need it, use it more than planned, or are afraid to live without it."

Even so, I don't want to give up alcohol, not entirely. So I've made certain rules. First, no drinking on an empty stomach. No more than two regulation-size drinks at a time. Nothing in the morning, ever. And I make sure that at least 2 days a week I have nothing to drink at all.

Will I be able to keep to it? I honestly don't know. But last night, when one son was blasting Lady Gaga's "Bad Romance" and the other was trying to weasel out of his homework to play a video game he calls "Kill, Kill, Kill," and my darling husband was trying to engage me in a discussion about lightbulbs, I stepped away from the bottle of vodka. I turned down the volume on Lady Gaga, confiscated the computer, and smiled and nodded through 20 minutes of lightbulb banter while simultaneously going to that happy place in my head.

But hey, I didn't have a drink.

"One new rule I've made: No more drinking on an empty stomach."

HEALTHY EATING WITH MICHELLE OBAMA

First lady Michelle Obama talks exclusively to Prevention *about how to get kids excited about eating healthy, her secret source of energy, and why women need to put themselves higher on their own priority lists.*

It's a typical day in the life of the White House. Outside, there's a rush of people on the wide, walking-friendly streets of DC. Inside, in the Map Room, we await our appointment with the first lady. Baroque molding frames the high-ceilinged, chalk-white room. Wainscoting, grandfather clocks, and a faded map circa 1800 adorn the walls. At every turn, stone-faced Secret Service staff walk by wordlessly in their standard-issue blue suits. A panoply of articulate, per-fect-postured young women in chic, simple dresses and heels, thumbing Black-Berrys held aloft, communicates urgent information in hushed tones. It's a formal place by casual Friday standards, but the brisk elegance, with its whiff of a bygone era, is somehow very reassuring.

Two doors down is the China Room; a noisy White House tour is held back from it with a simple red rope. It's a modest chamber, but its shelves are lined with startling objects: from Abraham Lincoln's perfectly preserved Limoges porcelain dating back to 1861 (heavy on purple tones and eagles) up through Roosevelt, Wilson, and beyond. It's impossible not to feel a flutter of history blowing lightly through the halls.

There is a sudden gathering of attention as the president's motorcade is leaving, heading to Andrews Air Force Base to fly to Pittsburgh and Orlando on his tour to try to rally support for the American Jobs Act.

Back in the Map Room, the appointed time is upon us. "She's coming!" someone whispers. The assembled make a U-shaped receiving line and check our posture. And then she is in: all upbeat vibe, easy laughter, and warm greetings (I remember you!), and the little bubble of tension is instantly popped. She is even leaner in person than she looks in photos, with a tiny waist and long legs.

After her portrait is taken, we travel through the East Colonnade to her peach-colored office for an interview. She gives a brief tour, pointing out photos of her daughters, Sasha and Malia, as well as her cherished collection of military coins nestled into slots in a felt display box, each one presented to her after a visit to a US military base.

And then it's time to talk about the second anniversary of what has become the signature platform of her tenure as first lady: Let's Move!, which encourages families and children to eat healthier fare and get more exercise, all in the service of fighting a growing epidemic of obesity.

"When we talk to parents, we talk about small changes for kids and about things that don't cost extra money."

Prevention: The economy is on everybody's mind, and in one sense, it's taking a toll on people's health, because people who have jobs are putting in more hours and therefore sleeping and exercising less. If they're not working, they're sleeping fitfully because they're worried.

First Lady Michelle Obama: The obesity rates among our kids have been going up for the past decade. So what we're seeing in terms of the effects on health isn't new and isn't unique to this economy. And the truth is that there's never a perfect time for good health and exercise. It's always difficult for families, no matter what their financial situation is, to figure out how to incorporate it, because that's simply not the habit of our culture.

"It's undeniable that what we eat and how much we move affect how we feel."

But clearly, this is a tough economic time, and a lot of families are hurting. So when we talk to parents, we talk about small changes for kids and things that don't cost extra money. Like adding water and eliminating sugary drinks and sodas. That's going to save money right there. Or adding a few more vegetables.

Another suggestion is to cook a meal, maybe not every night, but a couple more times a week than you usually do. That way you have leftovers, and you take your lunch to work. If people can find a way to slowly incorporate these changes into their lives, they're going to see the doctor less, and they'll have more energy, even in tough times of depression and struggle.

Prevention: When it comes to getting kids to exercise, what do you think is an acceptable bribe by parents to get kids to work out more?

Mrs. Obama: It's whatever motivates that kid. In my household, what motivates Sasha is very different from what motivates her big sister. It can be a television show they want to watch or an activity with a friend. But I try mostly to provide information to my kids about the why, because ultimately the bribe runs cold.

Prevention: Good way to put it. You've also talked about Sasha and Malia helping the White House chefs prep meals. What exactly do they like to do?

Mrs. Obama: Sasha always claimed not to like tomatoes, which is such a shame because we grow beautiful tomatoes out in our kitchen garden on the South Lawn. But then she took a cooking class at school where they made sandwiches with tomatoes, and all of a sudden she's saying how much she loves tomatoes. She insisted that the tomatoes she had at school were different. But the real difference is that she had put time into making that sandwich, so she was invested in it. And I think that's why involving kids in the cooking process is so important—they become invested, and they're willing to try new things, and they might discover that they actually like them.

Prevention: What are some healthy snacks that the girls specifically like?

Mrs. Obama: They both love dried and fresh fruit, and Sasha likes nuts. A few years ago, I always kept a bowl of fruit not just out on the countertop, but down low where they could reach it. That way, when they were running around from room to room, they could just grab a couple of grapes along the way, rather than pick up a cookie. That said, now they're older, so they do want cookies and ice cream like any other kids. The trick—and what we talk about—is not having those things every day.

Prevention: Our parent company, Rodale, publishes *Eat This, Not That!* And that brand is all about helping people understand the nutritional highs and lows of what they're buying in supermarkets and eating in restaurants. So we're interested to know if *Eat This, Not That!* has helped you and the president in your efforts.

Mrs. Obama: Tools and books like *Eat This, Not That!* are about giving people information, and the more information that families have to make better choices, the better off we are. Then each family can make the choices that make sense for them, because it is not a one-size-fits-all solution. No single family is alike; no single individual is alike.

Prevention: Once you start talking about eating healthy food, you very quickly get to the fact that our farms are riddled with pesticides, the seas are overfished, and we've made a host of environmental assaults against the planet. How much activism do we need to really change the conversation?

Mrs. Obama: We've got so much to do just to get people focused and informed. My motto is that you've got to take small chunks and go deep. I still think we have a lot of work to do just getting people to understand what we eat, how we eat, and how it's provided to us. Once you get people engaged and understanding that it's important to know what you eat and where it comes from, it just becomes a ripple effect on its own, because one thing leads to the next thing naturally. But right now, we're not even there with where you get your fish and how they're farmed. People don't know how much sodium and unhealthy fats are in processed foods. So I think we're still at the early stages of information, and we need to do more drilling down so that people get to those other places naturally, on their own.

Prevention: You touched on something that we think is incredibly relevant and important for American women, this double standard about weight and women. A University of Pennsylvania survey revealed that more than half of 620 doctors called their obese female patients awkward, ugly, and noncompliant. And more than a third of them called patients weak willed, sloppy, and lazy. What's your reaction?

Mrs. Obama: I would tell women: Forget about weight. Don't get on a scale. Stop measuring your waist. We can be upset about the double standard, but if we're teetering on the edge of unhealthy weights, that doesn't help us or our families. I look at it as setting an example. When I get up and work out, I'm working out just as much for my girls as I am for me, because I want them to see a mother who loves them dearly, who invests in them, but who also invests in herself. It's just as much about letting them know as young women that it is okay to put yourself a little higher on your priority list. It doesn't make you a selfish person. Men already feel just fine with an extra investment in themselves. And we encourage that.

But we have to turn that around for ourselves and show our young girls, I want you to be smart, I want you to be at the top of your class, I want you to play sports, I want you to sweat, I want you to run, I want you to eat right, and I want you to always do this. And I want you to teach your girls when you have them. I want us to pass that culture down. So I don't want us as women to get focused on these double standards. Let's just empower each other and get on it.

Prevention: Speaking of your workouts, you've said that your exercise regimen includes intervals of weight training and cardio, plus treadmill and some Pilates. Any update for us?

Mrs. Obama: I work out 6 or 7 days a week. But I do yoga now twice a week, because I'm beginning to notice as I get older that flexibility and mobility are critical.

Prevention: Do you and the president exercise at the same time?

Mrs. Obama: I usually get up to make sure that the girls get to school. And once they're out, I go up to work out.

He comes up afterward. So I'm usually in the middle of my workout when he's starting his.

Prevention: You start your day early, yes?

Mrs. Obama: I usually get up at 5:30. I either wait and get the girls out the door and go up to the gym after they leave. Or if I'm busy, I'll go right up to the gym and work out, because they're old enough now to set their own alarms and get themselves up.

Prevention: There is enormous pressure on women to look younger and stay looking younger for decades. Have you and your mom discussed this?

Mrs. Obama: Women are definitely under a lot of pressure, but I think it's important to remember that to look good, you have to feel good. I look at my mom at 76 and see how beautiful she looks and how wonderful she is with our daughters and with me and my husband, and I want that for myself when I'm her age. My mom also invests in herself more than when we were younger. She works out twice a week. She enjoys traveling with friends. She maintains a sensible diet. I've always said that

"I've always said that life gets good when you're 40 or 50."

life gets good when you're 40 or 50. And looking at my mom, I know that it just keeps getting better. So I hope I can follow her example and not just feel great at 76 years old but look great too.

Prevention: You've said that talking to your mom and girlfriends is your way of staying emotionally healthy. This is something *Prevention* readers say constantly too.

"I want my girls to see a mother who loves them dearly, who invests in them, but who also invests in herself."

Mrs. Obama: To be the best mom, the best wife, and the best friend and professional you can be, you have to take time for yourself. There's no negotiating that: We need to be higher up on our own priority list. For me, a key component of investing in myself is investing in my friendships and spending time with my girlfriends. I love my husband. He's the best partner I could ever wish for, and spending time with him is essential.

But it's also important to spend time with women. We reenergize each other, we support each other. And having those relationships does take time and investment, but it pays you back tenfold. To me, downloading with friends over lunch and going shopping with a girlfriend on the weekend are some of life's simple pleasures that lift you up at the end of a long day or week.

And that's a message I want to pass on to my girls too. You should invest in yourself, you should invest in your friendships, and that will give you the energy and happiness that we all need to be healthy and happy.

Prevention: Related to this, do people still underestimate the power of the mind-body connection? That a healthy emotional state leads to a healthy body and vice versa?

Mrs. Obama: We can't underestimate the link between health and happiness. It's hard to be happy if you're not feeling your best, and when you're feeling your best, it's much easier to make healthy choices.

Prevention: *Prevention* did a story about the fact that it's still legal in 37 states for insurance companies to charge women more money, which of course the Affordable Care Act will eliminate. The idea that women are penalized because they engage in preventive behaviors such as going for more checkups strikes us as outrageous.

Mrs. Obama: We have to make ourselves healthier because the cost of insurance and the way the systems work are so complicated that the best bet is to be healthy. That's the thing that we have the most control over: taking care of ourselves now.

Health reform is critical to prevention. But it's important for people to know that health reform is about fighting to ensure that people get preventive health care. The high rates of diabetes and strokes and heart attacks are all preventable with good access to medical care and preventive treatment. And nutrition is a part of that prevention. Many people don't have access to a nutritionist. Well, health care reform would allow that. It will mean that millions more people have access to the things that people with good insurance take for granted.

Prevention: Given how hard the president works and how much he cares, does it cause you pain when you see the president's approval ratings?

Mrs. Obama: I try not to pay too much attention to the polls. I like to stay focused on what my husband is achieving for our country, and I'm really proud of what he's been able to accomplish. If you look at what he's done on health care alone, it's really remarkable. He passed the Affordable Care Act, and because of that law, kids now get free preventive care, including healthy weight screenings. That's going to help us prevent obesity before it starts. It also means that women can receive preventive services such as mammograms without out-of-pocket costs. Those kinds of real changes are what's important to me, and I think to most Americans—what he's gotten done, not what the latest poll says.

STEPPING UP TO HEALTHIER EATING

First Lady Michelle Obama has made huge strides in getting Let's Move! principles put into practice in schools, supermarkets, and more. Here are some milestones to date.

FEBRUARY 9, 2010: Let's Move! launches, and school lunch suppliers pledge to reduce fat, sugar, and salt in their meals in the next 5 years, as well as double fruits and vegetables in 10 years.

MAY 17, 2010: Kraft Foods, Campbell Soup Company, and Kellogg Company agree to cut 1 trillion product calories by the end of 2012.

SEPTEMBER 14, 2010: With the President's Council on Fitness, Sports & Nutrition, the Million PALA Challenge asks for 1 million Americans to participate in physical activity 5 days a week. More than 1.7 million have enrolled.

SEPTEMBER 22, 2010: Kitchen equipment companies donate demonstration kits for 1,000 chefs working with schools to convince children that healthful food is better than junk food.

DECEMBER 13, 2010: President Obama signs the Healthy, Hunger-Free Kids Act, increasing access to healthy food for low-income children as well as funding for school meal programs.

MARCH 8, 2011: The United States Tennis Association commits to construct or renovate 3,000 kid-size tennis courts across the country.

JULY 20, 2011: Walmart, Supervalu, and others commit to develop 1,500 stores in "food deserts."

SEPTEMBER 15, 2011: Darden, owner of Olive Garden and Red Lobster, pledges to offer fruit, vegetables, and 1% milk with every kid's meal, plus reduce calories and sodium on regular menus.

OCTOBER 20, 2011: Let's Move! exceeds its goal, and the number of schools participating in the HealthierUS School Challenge is 2,161.

DECEMBER 12, 2011: Let's Move! Salad Bars to Schools delivers nearly 1,000 salad bars to schools, making fruits and vegetables accessible to thousands of kids.

Part 5

MIND
MATTERS

CHAPTER 22

YOUR DESIRE, DOUBLED

Call it a passion pep talk: The following five words will bring you closer in the bedroom.

When a relationship is new, lovemaking feels as natural and spontaneous as sunrise. Sex just seems to happen. But after years of marriage, mortgages, and maternity leave, it can fall off the Things I'm Dying to Do list and join the Things I Really Ought to Do list—right under "start diet" and "flood-proof kids' rooms." You know you're always purring with happiness when you do have a romantic romp with your partner, but finding the time, energy, and even the desire can become elusive.

According to a new Australian study, 27 percent of wives and 54 percent of husbands say they would like to have more sex. But 22 percent of married women in their fifties and 37.9 percent of married women in their sixties haven't had sex during the past year. To bridge this desire gap, we consulted top psychologists and sex experts to share their insights for bringing back that loving feeling. Not surprisingly, it starts with what you think and what you say to each other. Here are five fire-starting words to help boost your sexual mood.

PASSION PEP TALK #1

Now?

"I like to fool around in the evening, but my husband's a morning man. When we didn't have kids or demanding jobs, it was easier. Is there any way to synchronize our sexual watches?"

First, make sure you understand the reasons you each prefer a different time of day. Is it because he's too exhausted and agitated after a day at work? Are you distracted in the morning about getting the kids off to school?

"After you've identified your concerns, it's up to the other person to come up with a practical solution," says Terri Orbuch, PhD, a psychologist and the author of *5 Simple Steps to Take Your Marriage from Good to Great*. Maybe you can arrange for the kids to have a sleepover with Grandma once a week if she lives nearby. Maybe your husband can work on putting his office politics obsession on ice for one night.

If the logistics still can't be managed, make like preschoolers and take turns.

"If you each compromise on timing, you'll see that it makes you appreciate your partner's consideration more," Dr. Orbuch says. "Once you get your body started on a sexual course, your brain and mood will soon catch up."

PASSION PEP TALK #2

More!

"Although I reach orgasm most easily through oral sex, my husband seems to oblige me only grudgingly. How can I get him to be more into it?"

You have more wind at your back here than you realize, advises Debby Herbenick, PhD, a research scientist in the Applied Health Science department at Indiana University. A recent Kinsey Institute study of middle-age couples found that one of the most important predictors of a man's happiness in a relationship was his ability to make his partner climax. So if you make it clear that this particular technique is your ticket to the top, he's likely to cooperate.

"Try saying, 'I get really turned on when you do this, and I'd love you to do it more often,'" says Andrea Syrtash, the author of *Cheat on Your Husband (with Your Husband)*. Also, don't assume he's begrudging you; maybe he's a little insecure about his performance, Dr. Orbuch says. Again, he'll probably appreciate specific feedback, and few things are more of a turn-on for a man than watching a woman become turned on. Finally, suggest any changes that might make oral sex more appealing to him, like trimming your pubic hair or trying a new position that's more comfortable for him.

"A give-and-take is the best way to remove any defensiveness and get him to open up," Dr. Herbenick says.

PASSION PEP TALK #3

Hello.

"When we've been fighting, I don't feel like having sex, but he's as hot to trot whether we've just had a nice dinner out in a restaurant or spent all evening arguing about our kitchen renovation."

Some stereotypes about men and women are true, and this is one of them.

"Men seek sex as a way to feel close, but women need to feel close in order to have sex," Dr. Orbuch says.

After an argument, women often get trapped in their heads, replaying the details of the disagreement and dwelling on the negative emotions. In fact, according to a recent study in the *Journal of Family Psychology*, women actually derive relationship satisfaction if their partners know they're upset, because women take it as a sign that their husbands are trying to empathize with them and really do want to be attentive (even though it might be just perceived effort). Contrast that with men, who see sex as completely separate from whatever else is going on in the marriage, and it's clear to see how friction emerges—and remains.

So how do you find common ground? First, put a lid on the verbal zingers and change your script.

"Research shows that healthy relationships have five positive interactions for every negative one," Syrtash says.

With that ratio in mind, she recommends committing to 10 minutes a day of quality communication to counteract the bedroom buzzkill of daily disputes and distractions. Each day, incorporate as little as 5 to 10 minutes during which certain topics, such as in-laws, children, and housework, are off the table. This might feel a little forced at first, but stick with it, and you'll find that you'll fill up your bank of affection—which will not only help you navigate through disagreements but also enhance your emotional and physical intimacy.

PASSION PEP TALK #4

Wow!

"Since I've gained weight, I feel self-conscious. Plus, I haven't been working out as much as I should. Short of a makeover, how can I recapture my confidence in bed?"

It's not how you look that matters. It's how you feel about how you look.

"Studies have shown that body image has nothing to do with actual appearance," Dr. Herbenick says. "No matter how 'lumpy' you're feeling, it's the ability to manage your anxieties about your body that makes the difference."

Think outside the Sofia Vergara box. Plenty about your body is sexy: It's not always a wasp-thin waistline or Barbie-doll breasts.

"Take a good look at your sculpted shoulders or graceful neck," Syrtash says. According to studies conducted at the UCLA School of Medicine, redirecting your thoughts toward something more positive—a process called neuroplasti-

WHY BEDROOM BOLDNESS IS BETTER

Women are more likely than men to try out new sexual activities—and are more satisfied as a result, according to sex researcher Kristen Mark, PhD. In a recent survey of more than 3,000 adults by goodinbed.com, Dr. Mark says, she found that "women had engaged in more adventurous bedtime exploits than men, and those who experimented with talking dirty, stripping for a lover, or leaving the lights on during sex reported feeling very fulfilled by the sexual experience." Start by sharing a fantasy with your partner, and let the fun unfurl.

city—actually rewires the neural connections in your brain that relay messages. That sort of self-talk can help reinforce sexual thoughts, and then it's a matter of nature taking its course.

PASSION PEP TALK #5

Yes!

"After 13 years of marriage, I still very much love my husband. But I don't feel as much desire as I'd like to."

"Low libido is both a common and complex issue," says Tieraona Low Dog, MD, of the Arizona Center for Integrative Medicine and the author of *Life Is Your Best Medicine*. "Hormones can wreak havoc in lots of ways. Birth control pills are known for decreasing testosterone and therefore diminishing sex drive at any age—even well into your forties—as do low thyroid function and the hormone swings that are hallmarks of perimenopause and full-blown menopause."

If these aren't issues for you, then it's probably those old standby passion derailers when there's no particular problem: stress and worry.

But there are terrific natural aphrodisiacs that can help. Dr. Low Dog recommends three in particular, starting with shatavari, which is derived from wild asparagus.

"Its Sanskrit name means 'she who possesses 100 husbands,' and while its primary use is for hot flashes, it also aids libido and fertility," Dr. Low Dog says. Another example is maca, considered a passion plant in its native Peru. "Damiana is also worth trying, either as a capsule or liqueur," she says. "Drink 1 ounce after dinner and give your husband a shot."

"Plenty about your body is sexy."

You'll be saying yes in no time.

CHAPTER 23

THE PICTURE OF HEALTH

This remarkable group impressed us most with their commitment to healthy living—against all odds. Read on for the inspiring lessons they can teach all of us.

Do you live a healthy life? Have you overcome a personal challenge? Do you inspire others? We asked these questions when we kicked off our annual Picture of Health contest with the CBS television show *The Doctors*. As we pored over the hundreds of heartwarming entries, the following five men and women stood out for their can-do spirit and commitment to helping others. Read their moving stories.

"MOTIVATING SICK KIDS KEEPS ME STRONG TOO"

Chris Word, 52, Los Angeles

Two of the biggest turning points in Chris Word's life occurred while he was wandering hallways. First, that's how he got the lifesaving treatment that helped him beat his battle with stage 3 colon cancer. Diagnosed years after he started experiencing symptoms such as bleeding, Word was told he needed major surgery that would require removing his sphincter muscle (and a lifetime of wearing a colonoscopy bag).

Word, a father of six, insisted on finding someone who would save his quality of life. He went to the best hospital he could think of and paced the halls until he met a surgeon who would rethink his case.

When Word woke up from surgery with 18 inches of his colon gone (but sphincter still intact), he felt thankful—and reenergized. Inspired by all the child cancer patients he met while walking the corridors during recovery (the second milestone moment), Word felt driven to have some good come of his cancer bout. So he started the Lifedriven Foundation, a nonprofit that supports cancer research and treats children battling the disease with trips to Disneyland.

"There is so much about cancer that people have no control over, but we can give a family a moment in time to experience some joy," Word says.

He outfitted a van with the Lifedriven logo and drives around to share his story. "I love telling people how that dollar they give is going to make a child smile," he says.

HEALTHY HABITS

Picture of health Chris Word says he does the following every day.

OVERDOSE ON VEGETABLES. I can't believe how many greens I eat now. My wife makes me have a vegetable at every meal.

MAKE PEOPLE LAUGH. When someone else is smiling, I feel happier too.

WAKE UP AND FEEL GRATEFUL. Whether it's raining, snowing, or the most gorgeous day ever, I don't have anything to be sad about.

"I feel healthiest when I'm out driving my van and telling people about my charity work, because that means I'm helping kids," says Word.

"I STARTED A RUNNING CLUB FOR STUDENTS"

Paula Bruchhaus, 43, Lake Charles, Louisiana

Completing a marathon is the best feeling in the world for Paula Bruchhaus. But it's a recent emotion for the schoolteacher and mother of two, who spent more than 35 years trying to shake off her childhood nickname, Stump ("because I was short and round"). In 2002, after watching her husband successfully slim down, Bruchhaus followed suit—eventually losing 80 pounds. She ditched buffets and the school cafeteria and prepared meals at home. She ran on the treadmill or attended Spinning class at the gym every morning, where she developed a new love of exercise that she couldn't help but pass on to her fourth graders.

Her classroom became adorned with trophies and medals. (Bruchhaus grew passionate about races; she's done eight marathons and a full Ironman triathlon.) She saw how interested her kids were in her hobby. When she heard of a kids' triathlon, she encouraged students to sign up. After she saw how much fun they had—and how eager parents seemed to help their children get active—Bruchhaus knew she could do something more to help her school stay healthy.

That something became Prien Lake Elementary School's first running club. The kids run at home after school and on weekends, and they log their miles in a chart their parents sign. Bruchhaus raised money from local businesses for T-shirts and prizes. For every mile, kids get a sticker. For every 25, they receive a prize such as a yo-yo or a lunch box. Students were soon running in local races, joining physical activity with philanthropy. Over the years, her students have raised $25,000 for charity.

"The club is also about finishing what you start and pushing yourself even when you don't feel like it," says Bruchhaus.

Last year, Bruchhaus was promoted to physical education teacher, where she continues to inspire the entire school.

"I help kids love exercise."
—Paula Bruchhaus

Picture of health Paula Bruchhaus does these things every day.

WAKE UP EARLY. I love going to the gym first thing. This also makes me less likely to overeat because I don't want to ruin what I've already accomplished.

MAKE EXERCISE FUN. I try to make gym class all about playing games.

EAT A HEALTHY BREAKFAST. I used to have bowls of sugary cereal. Now I have Egg Beaters omelets, low-fat cheese, and fruit.

"Gym used to be my least favorite part of the day. It's where I felt inferior," she says. "So I make sure my students feel happy and confident." On the first day of school, she shows students photos from her past. "I explain that we're not all going to be super fast or strong, but our goal is simply to improve. It is possible to change simply by eating healthy and exercising."

"I feel healthiest when I cross a finish line of a triathlon or race. I literally feel like superwoman the rest of the day," says Puala Bruchhaus.

"I PROVE BOUNCING BACK IS IN YOUR ATTITUDE"

Dawn Forgione, 51, Delray Beach, Florida

If she hits a bump in the road, Dawn Forgione has one response: Keep going. In 2006, she endured serious injuries, including 40 stitches to her face and knocked-out teeth, after a bad bicycle spill while training for a 150-mile charity ride. That's just the tip of the unlucky-in-health iceberg for Forgione, who works as a real estate agent in South Florida and lives with one of her two 20-something daughters. Her issues read like a laundry list—bouts of cervical dysplasia, endometriosis that led to four laparoscopies and ultimately a radical hysterectomy at 41, knee surgery, two recent hip replacements, skin cancer, and breast cancer followed by a lumpectomy and radiation.

But Forgione is not one to mope around with a "Why me?" attitude. Just a

few days after going home from the hospital following her violent bike crash, Forgione went back to
work.

*"I'm so proud to say
I'm a survivor."*

—Dawn Forgione

"Everyone thought I was crazy with my face so
banged up, but life goes on."

Instead of being upset about her hysterectomy, she felt grateful that she was
pain free. Forgione also credits her resiliency to her healthy life. She hits the
gym for Zumba classes, strength-training, and cardio. She eats a lot of fruit,
salad, and grilled chicken and salmon.

Forgione infuses her get-up-and-keep-going mentality into all of the groups
she's helped through the years, such as the American Cancer Society, the Children's Cancer Caring Center in Miami, and the March of Dimes. She's also
started grassroots efforts: organizing a Thanksgiving dinner for special-needs
adults and a volunteer group to paint homes. Among the healthy habits
that Forgione promotes are (1) always wear a bike helmet and (2) get regular
screenings. Both her breast and skin cancers were detected during routine
tests.

"I love to be a positive role model and show others that a diagnosis is not a
death sentence," she says.

"I feel healthiest when my mind is happy and I'm thinking of something joyful. Health starts at the top and trickles down. Your mental health has so much
to do with your physical health," says Forgione.

HEALTHY HABITS

Every day Dawn Forgione does these things.

REFLECT ON THE GOOD THINGS IN MY LIFE—when I get dressed in the
morning and right before I go to sleep.

NEVER SAY THE WORD PROBLEM. I hate that word; I always say challenge,
which helps me resolve an issue and move on.

DO SOMETHING PHYSICAL EVERY DAY. When I can't go to the gym, I take my
dog for an extralong walk or do situps and stretches.

THE PICTURE OF HEALTH 257

"I TEACH OTHERS TO BE CLEANER AND GREENER"

Kristi Marsh, 39, North Easton, Massachusetts

When Kristi March felt a lump in her right breast while taking a shower, her entire life changed. A whirlwind of appointments and health decisions ensued, leading to a diagnosis of stage 3 breast cancer, followed by a mastectomy and rounds of chemo, Herceptin, and radiation. Married with three children ages 7 and younger, the then-35-year-old Marsh refused to let cancer get in the way of her life. She skated with her daughter after chemo and camped by the ocean with her family during the summer when she received radiation. Grateful for all the support she received, she wanted to give something back to her community. She organized a fund-raising dinner with friends that raised $40,000 in the name of the Dana-Farber Cancer Institute.

Marsh says cancer taught her two things. The first: to step outside her usual comfort zones.

"In Hollywood's version of cancer, they don't really show that your eyebrows and eyelashes disappear too, and you still have to grocery shop," Marsh says. "That's real life. The kids still need you."

The second lesson continues to transform her life and also those of others in her community. While undergoing treatment, Marsh was amazed by her body's ability to heal.

"I realized that our bodies try so hard to survive and overcome, but we often compromise that with unhealthy choices that increase our exposure to pesticides, hormones, antibiotics, and pollutants."

She researched nontoxic products and joined a CSA (community supported agriculture) farm, on which her family volunteers often. Marsh even started raising her own hens for organic eggs.

"I've totally transformed how I feed my family and how my kids view food," she says. "Now it's not just something that arrives from the store in a can or box but a learning experience."

"I inspire others to live cleaner, greener lives."
—Kristi Marsh

Friends and neighbors became curious about her clean-living efforts, so Marsh started an educational organization called Choose Wiser. Through intimate workshops, she shares her tips with local groups.

"I felt like there was a gap between all the information that's out there and what busy moms are supposed to do about it," she says. "I hope to educate people about what fits best into their lives so they can make healthy changes."

"I feel healthiest when I combine exercise, nature, and exploration, such as hiking in a state park. That's just pure joy for me," says Marsh.

"I AM A WEIGHT-LOSS INSPIRATION FOR OTHERS"

Linda Goff, 42, Rolla, Missouri

After her insurance company told her in 2003 that she was "too healthy" for gastric bypass, Linda Goff was crushed. The 300-pound working mom of two boys thought surgery would be a quick fix. Then she got angry and decided that gaining more weight would get the procedure approved. For 4 years, Goff ate whatever she wanted, dressed in the dark, and avoided mirrors.

"I can't believe what a horrible example I was setting for my kids," she says.

Most upsetting, the weight-gain bender was taking a huge toll on her marriage, one of the great joys of her life.

"It was unfair of me to expect my husband to find me attractive when I was doing so many deliberately unhealthy things," Goff says.

One day, it became clear that the intimacy with her husband was fading fast, and she didn't want her marriage to become a platonic friendship. "I broke

"I lost 160 pounds to get healthy and save my marriage."
—Linda Goff

down and prayed for the strength, courage, and patience to take the first step."

A switch flipped, and Goff began the little changes that helped her lose 160 pounds and shrink from a size 26 to 6. She tracked calories and aimed for 2,000 a day—half of what she'd been consuming—and took hikes with her Labradoodle. Buoyed by support from her husband, family, and friends, Goff dropped 100 pounds, and then joined a gym—a lesson in conquering fear.

"The gym can be very intimidating, but this time I refused to be embarrassed," she says.

Today, Goff feels better than she did at 25, and she helps counsel weight-loss support groups at a hospital, gym, and church. "I want to let people know that good choices are just like bad ones. They can become lifelong habits too."

"I feel healthiest when I'm shopping for clothes! Okay, that sounds vain, but I love the real-world proof that I'm a healthy size," says Goff.

HEALTHY HABITS

Picture of health Linda Goff recommends these everyday habits.

REFUSE TO HAVE REGRETS. I think of my past failures as practice runs for the journey I'm on now.

CHEERLEAD OTHERS. I mentor a group of people I've met through the hospital on their weight-loss journeys. We help keep each other in check. I view it as a loving kick in the pants.

THANK GOD. My faith gave me the courage to take the first step when I failed so many times before. And God gave me awesome family and friends who love me and keep me accountable.

TWO "BAD" HABITS THAT ARE GOOD FOR YOU

Can't kick your snickerdoodle addiction? Spend too much time on Facebook? Some "vices" you've long assumed were naughty or simply unproductive can actually offer pretty nice health perks, as long as you don't overdo it. See if you can guess the surprising answers to the following questions: Which "bad" habit...

BOOSTS BRAINPOWER AND CURBS CRAVINGS?

1. Having a smoke
2. Eating a T-bone
3. Chewing gum
4. Sniffing a cleaning solvent

ANSWER: 3. Chewing gum boosts thinking and alertness in part by increasing blood flow to the brain, finds a new study. Research shows that people who chew sugarless gum before eating have fewer sweet cravings and eat about 36 fewer calories, says Judy Caplan, RD, an Academy of Nutrition and Dietetics spokesperson.

HELPS EASE ALLERGIES?

1. Living like a slob
2. Swimming right after eating
3. Biting your fingernails
4. Eating 8 ounces of processed cheese

ANSWER: 1. Not being a total neat freak may help you breathe easier. A Kingston University study found that dust mites, which can cause hay-feverlike symptoms and even trigger asthma attacks in some people, were less able to survive in messy, unmade beds because conditions were too warm and dry for them.

CHAPTER 24

2-MINUTE STRESS SOLUTIONS

New findings in neuroscience, nutrition, and psychology reveal the fastest ways to reduce tension and actually change your brain and body for the better.

When we were 5, we might have sucked our thumbs for stress relief. As adults, many of us self-soothe with junk food, a glass (or two) of wine and maybe some mindless TV. But those are fixes that don't actually fix anything.

Luckily, recent studies reveal some easy ways to lift your spirits and lower your stress that actually create positive shifts in your brain and body.

"Stress triggers the release of the hormone cortisol, which can damage our brains and weaken our cardiovascular and immune systems over time," says neuropsychologist Rick Hanson, PhD, the author of *Buddha's Brain*. We asked experts for their best instant mood boosters, backed by the latest research in nutrition, psychology, and neuroscience. Follow these tips, and you'll be saying "aah" in no time.

PUT ON A HAPPY FACE

Try this simple, instantaneous stress reliever: Smile. A recent study from the University of Kansas found that making a happy face whenever you're upset or tense can actually reduce your body's response to stress and leave you feeling more relaxed.

Another study, this one at the University of Wisconsin, found that people who'd had Botox injections were less prone to anger because they couldn't express it. What's the lesson? Just fake it till you make it.

THINK: HOT HANDS

When fear and anxiety take hold, the nervous system directs blood flow to the largest muscles, an evolutionary response to protect against physical danger. This redirected flow often results in cold hands. So when you warm them, that automatically signals your nervous system that it's okay to calm down, says neuropsychologist Marsha Lucas, PhD.

"Even simply visualizing warm hands can be enough to help turn off the fight-or-flight reaction," she says.

DONATE SOME DOLLARS

Giving money to a good cause makes you feel better than buying a pair of designer jeans—and studies prove that this is true, say Elizabeth Dunn, PhD, of the University of British Columbia, and Michael Norton, PhD, of Harvard Business School.

Plus, you don't have to be a millionaire to enjoy this karmic boost. The researchers learned that those who gave even $5 to someone else felt measurably better than those who bought themselves a treat instead.

LOAD UP ON WHOLE GRAINS

"If you're feeling grumpy, the best idea is to eat an all-carb whole grain snack, and you should feel happier within a half hour," says nutritionist Elizabeth

Somer, RD, the author of *Eat Your Way to Sexy.* "The carbs raise blood sugar, which boosts serotonin, a neurotransmitter associated with calm, positive feelings that last."

Aim for 30 grams of carbs: 4 cups of air-popped popcorn or half of a whole wheat English muffin (but not a bag of Chips Ahoy) will do the trick, Somer advises.

DIG IN THE DIRT

According to a 2011 Dutch study published in the *Journal of Health Psychology,* 30 minutes of gardening reduces stress levels more effectively than 30 minutes of reading quietly in a room. The researchers say it's the result of the physical activity.

But perhaps the secret lies in the dirt itself. A few studies have shown a link between a common bacterium (*M. vaccae*) found in garden soil and increased serotonin levels, meaning less anxiety and better concentration. Gardeners might inhale this bacterium while digging in the soil.

NATURAL SOOTHERS

We asked *Prevention* editorial board member Tieraona Low Dog, MD, the author of *Life Is Your Best Medicine*, for her favorite herbal stress soothers.

"I call milky oat seed tincture 'meditation in a bottle.' Just 2 to 3 milliliters instantly relaxes you," Dr. Low Dog says. She also suggests drinking tea with kava, a South Pacific herb with a powerful settling effect.

"Lemon, lime, and orange scents are all known to lift your spirits," she says. Dissolve 15 drops of one of those essential oils in 2 tablespoons of water and pour into a spray bottle for a pick-me-up. Before bed, mist your pillow with a lavender oil spritz.

GIVE YOURSELF A HUG

When you think negatively about yourself, the brain's amygdala sends signals that increase blood pressure and raise adrenaline and cortisol levels. Researcher Kristin Neff, PhD, at the University of Texas, recommends the "surreptitious self-hug"—wrapping your arms around yourself and squeezing. Even your own touch releases oxytocin and other biochemicals that promote well-being.

FOCUS ON THE EXHALE

We've all heard that deep breathing is crucial to feeling tranquil, but the most important part of it is breathing out, Dr. Hanson says: "When you elongate your exhalations, you spark your parasympathetic nervous system, which slows down your heart rate." Take three long exhalations, making them twice as long as your inhalation.

JUST MOVE IT—A LITTLE

John Ratey, MD, a Harvard Medical School professor and the author of *Spark: The Revolutionary New Science of Exercise and the Brain*, says just 2 minutes of exercise is enough to change your mood, as long as you raise your heart rate.

"Anything from squats to jumping jacks supplies a surge of neurotransmitters, such as norepinephrine, dopamine, and serotonin—the same targets as antidepressants," he says.

EXERCISE WITH A FRIEND

The benefits of having a friend join you when you exercise go beyond the moral support you need to go the distance. Just having that company might also soothe you. Researchers at Santa Clara and Stanford Universities have found that exercising with a partner enhances a workout's stress-reducing effects—a boon for body and mind.

Subjects who sweated it out with a partner felt calmer than solo exercisers did immediately following their workout and even later that night. Huffing and puffing through an uphill ride? You don't have to worry about talking. Whether or not the subjects chatted during the activity did not change their results.

SIMPLE STRESS RELIEVERS

According to a meQuilibrium.com survey, 73 percent of us are often frustrated by "the little things." Keep calm and carry on with the following tips from meQuilibrium's chief science officer, Andrew Shatte, PhD.

THIS HAPPENS	YOU FEEL	TRY THIS
Your boss made so many notes on a presentation, you're sure you'll be fired	Anxious. You wake up at 3 a.m. convinced you'll soon be living in a dumpster.	Write your fears in a notebook. Reexamine them in the light of day so you have a clearer idea of what actions to take.
A friend asks you to dog-sit, but you're too busy, so you say no.	Guilty. You spend hours wondering if you should have just said yes.	Take guilt to task. Ask yourself what you really owe this person. Would you expect her to drop everything for you?
Someone cuts ahead of you in line at the deli.	Angry! Does he not see you? How can he be so rude?	We all think life should be fair, but very often it isn't. Resolve not to let a careless act ruin your day.
Your Thai take-out order arrives and is wrong. Again.	Depressed. Bad luck seems to follow you everywhere.	Mistakes happen. It doesn't mean you live under a dark cloud. Take action: Call to ask for a free pad thai next time.

BE A JAW DROPPER

"Relaxing your tongue and jaw sends a message to your brain stem and limbic system to turn off the stress hormones adrenaline and cortisol," says Dr. Lucas. Simply let your tongue go limp in your mouth, and then open your mouth slightly, which will instantly loosen up your jaw. "These exercises help bring our parasympathetic nervous system online, which tells our bodies to rest and restore," Dr. Lucas says.

THINK SENSUALLY

Next time you're feeling frazzled, try a tactile solution. During peak moments of stress, endorphins released into the brain relieve pain and begin a recovery period. Doing things that feel good physically—such as taking a warm shower or listening to a favorite piece of music—mimics this process and shuts down the stress deluge.

FATTEN UP THAT LATTE

When stress makes you unfocused, caffeine's stimulating qualities might promote a can-do attitude.

"To supersize that good feeling, drink your coffee with a little bit of organic whole milk instead of fat free. The extra protein and fat make you feel more satiated and therefore calmer," says Drew Ramsey, MD, an assistant professor of psychiatry at Columbia University.

NIBBLE ON CHOCOLATE

"A Johns Hopkins University study found that the taste of sweetness on your tongue causes a surge of feel-good endorphins," Somer says.

Also, dark chocolate has compounds called flavonoids that also affect mood: According to a 2010 study published in the *Journal of Psychopharmacology*, cocoa flavonoids improved both mental acuity and attitude.

Additionally, in a 2009 study by the *American Chemical Society*, eating a mere 1.4 ounces of dark chocolate daily lowered stress hormone levels. The key is to limit yourself to just a few bites, because the sugar in chocolate can cause a crash later.

"Plus, when you binge on anything, your blood is diverted to your gut away from your brain and muscles, which leaves you feeling tired," Somer says.

BEEF UP

A burger isn't all bad, as long as it's made from grass-fed beef. That's because pastured beef is high in conjugated linoleic acid, which is a fat that fights cancer and belly fat and has also been shown to protect brain cells from worry, Dr. Ramsey says. Grass-fed beef also supplies a good dose of iron, which might boost your energy levels.

"As many as 15 percent of women ages 20 to 40 are iron deficient, and most iron-deficient people are tired and stressed," Dr. Ramsey says.

WASH AWAY YOUR WORRIES

Lady Macbeth tried this centuries ago, but new research confirms that washing your hands for at least 20 seconds can rinse away your troubles.

"Because we associate being 'moral' with being 'clean,' washing can have the surprising effect of removing negative psychological residue too," says Spike W. S. Lee, a coauthor of the study.

CHAPTER 25

FIRST EVER! *PREVENTION'S* HEALTHY TV AWARDS

Take some much-needed me-time and catch up on some of our favorite shows!

We watched 'em, we rated 'em, and here are our picks for shows that deliver the best messages and role models for healthier lifestyles.

HEALTHY TV WINNERS

These are our *Prevention* top picks.

Hot In Cleveland, TV Land: Three witty women (Wendie Malick, Jane Leeves, and Valerie Bertinelli) adopt Cleveland as the heartland of self-acceptance to show that hot equals healthy. *Hot in Cleveland*'s divas are all 50 and over—and fabulous! The 91-year-old spark plug Betty White adds to the high jinks.

The Biggest Loser, NBC: This show is a phenomenon, driving contestants to get healthy and drop pounds so they can win $250,000. With the help of trainer Jillian Michaels and host Alison Sweeney, these men and women touch viewers' hearts and minds as they reshape their bodies—and their lives.

Parks and Recreation, NBC: Amy Poehler heads a cast that's fun, funny, and sexy. When Chris (Rob Lowe) offers a guest some greens and purrs, "Try it, salad's good for you," you know mesclun's made it to the big time.

Dancing with the Stars, ABC, and *So You Think You Can Dance,* FOX: On *Dancing with the Stars* (hosted by Brooke Burke and Tom Bergeron), stars like Kirstie Alley have made dancing for weight loss simply inspiring. And *So You Think You Can Dance* has given us congressionally endorsed National Dance Day, which

HOLD THE APPLAUSE

FEMALE JOGGER DOWN!

Body of Proof, ABC: We were bummed when, in a time-honored TV tradition, yet another female jogger dropped dead, this one from downing a poisoned sports drink while out for a solo run. Note to writers: Leave the runners alone!

THUMBS-DOWN TO BOTTOMS UP

Cougar Town, ABC: It's one thing to have a glass or two of wine, but *Cougar Town*'s giant goblet—dubbed Big Carl by Courteney Cox's character, Jules—holds a bottle and a half of vino, which she glugs almost every episode. Put a warning label on it, guys.

WORST MISSED HEALTH OPPORTUNITY

NCIS, CBS: Actor Sean H. Murray got the Twittersphere chirping with concern over his dramatic weight loss. So why didn't NCIS take advantage and have his character, Agent Timothy McGee, gab a bit about his new diet plan?

promotes an active lifestyle. Let's tango!

The Dr. Oz Show, syndicated: By taking the mystery out of the medical and adding showmanship and sex appeal, Mehmet Oz, MD, is making America healthier, one episode at a time. With the help of wacky props and an "Assistant of the Day," he gets viewers to improve their lives.

BEST INTEGRATION OF MEDICAL NEWS

Grey's Anatomy, ABC: This hospital drama, starring Ellen Pompeo and Patrick Dempsey, has fearlessly tackled tough, topical health issues with intelligence and compassion, from Alzheimer's disease to post-traumatic stress, ever since the show's inception in 2005.

MOST SENSITIVE PORTRAYAL OF AUTISM

Parenthood, NBC: Watching Adam and Kristina Braverman (Peter Krause and Monica Potter) come to terms with their son Max's special needs gave a heartfelt—and helpful—glimpse of families living with a loved one with a condition on the autism spectrum.

MOST CLEVER HEALTHY-LIFESTYLE CUES

Rizzoli & Isles, TNT: Detective Rizzoli (Angie Harmon) and her partner Dr. Isles (Sasha Alexander) might be crime-fighting babes, but they never waste an opportunity to slip health information into a sentence—chastising a colleague to switch to decaf coffee or owning up to a childhood as an overweight kid, for example.

MOST RELEVANT USE OF A MEDICAL BREAKTHROUGH

Glee, FOX: This ensemble musical show (with Jane Lynch, Matthew Morrison, and Lea Michele) has a ton of heart, featuring a wheelchair-bound character as just one of the gang. When Artie (Kevin McHale) got outfitted with a robotic exoskeleton called ReWalk, which (in real life) allows paraplegics partial mobility, we all got lumps in our throats.

BEST INTEGRATION OF GREEN LIVING

Modern Family, ABC: Typical episodes include Mitchell (Jesse Tyler Ferguson) coming home from shopping for local produce at the farmers' market, his reusable market basket filled with kale, while the Dunphys (Julie Bowen and Ty Burrell) play a boys-versus-girls ball game for the right to pass on the day's dishwashing duty.

BEST WINDOW INTO THE AGING GUY'S SOUL

Men of a Certain Age, TNT: Whether it's adjusting to reading glasses or coping with bigger-deal scares such as cancer, Ray Romano and his band of buds give women a secret decoder ring to men's mental and physical health concerns.

MOST DARING CONCEPT

The Big C, SHOWTIME: Skin cancer takes center stage as actress Laura Linney's Cathy lives a full life, despite her diagnosis.

SPECIAL MENTIONS

We'd like to give a shout-out to the following shows, which we believe deserve extra attention.

THE ADVOCACY AWARD: Mariska Hargitay takes her *Law & Order: SVU* character's job so seriously that she created the Joyful Heart Foundation to help victims of sexual assault, domestic violence, and child abuse.

THE NEWSMAKERS AWARD: To *Today's* Natalie Morales, whose marathon run roused viewers to better fitness; *Today's* Hoda Kotb and *Good Morning America's* Robin Roberts for sensitively bringing to bear their own experiences with breast cancer; Elisabeth Hasselbeck, who uses *The View* to share the struggles of celiac disease; and *Kelly Ripa*, the fund- and awareness-raiser for the Ovarian Cancer Research Fund.

THE SOUL FOODIES AWARD: To Giada De Laurentiis, who proves that you can enjoy healthy home cooking; Ellie Krieger, RD, who shows that eating smart can be tasty too; and *Iron Chef's* Cat Cora, for cooking healthy under pressure.

CHAPTER 26

SLEEP LIKE A BABY TONIGHT

Get snoozing with this science-backed program that's been bed-tested on real women. Bonus: You could drop 2 pounds a week.

If the sound of your alarm clock makes you want to cry, scream, or throw something (we've been there too), it's time to stop spending your days groggy and grumpy, grab your sneaks, and get moving. Now, we know what you're thinking: But I'm too tired to exercise! Before you toss this book aside, however, give us a moment to explain.

Research shows that regular aerobic exercise, such as a brisk walk or a heart-pumping Zumba class, can make it easier to fall asleep faster and stay asleep longer. Yoga has also been shown to be an all-natural sleep aid. A study published in the *Indian Journal of Medical Research* found that insomniacs who practiced yoga for 6 months fell asleep 10 minutes faster, slept an hour longer, and woke up feeling more refreshed than insomniacs who didn't practice yoga.

Of course, all that lab research doesn't mean a thing if it doesn't work in the real world of work deadlines, financial worries, changing hormones, and a slew of other variables that can make it difficult to sleep soundly. So to see if adding a little sweat to a daily routine would really help the average 40-plus woman sleep better, we asked 15 previously sedentary and sleep-deprived women to put the theory to the test. The youngest was 40; the oldest, 64. Their challenge: Aim to do 30 minutes of moderate to vigorous aerobic activity five times a week, as well as a few relaxing yoga poses before bed, for 5 weeks.

And guess what? It worked. At the start of the program, the women had trouble either falling asleep or staying asleep—or both. Four of them took over-the-counter sleep aids regularly. At the end of the program, everyone was sleeping more soundly on a regular basis. They found it easier to fall asleep and stay asleep naturally, with fewer wakeful periods during the night. Even 64-year-old Lorenda Murr, who had taken prescription and OTC sleep aids for more than 8 years, slept well. As a bonus, the women had more energy. Each lost an average of 7 pounds and 8 inches. Some women dropped as much as 9 or 10 pounds.

"I've had trouble staying asleep ever since going through early menopause at age 37," says Dana Dornburgh, 41, a high school guidance counselor in Holland Patent, New York. "It was normal for me to go to bed at midnight, lie awake from about 2 until 4, and then get up for work at 6 a.m. I was exhausted all the time and reached for sugary snacks such as chocolate to get through the day. But once I started exercising, I began sleeping consistently through the night. I have also dropped 6 pounds, feel great, and no longer find myself craving an energy boost from candy."

EXERCISE HELPED REAL WOMEN SCORE MORE SHUT-EYE

Laurie Schmidt, 53, an ad designer in Siren, Wisconsin, used to wake up 12 to 18 times throughout the night, sometimes lying awake and watching the clock for up to an hour.

"It was awful. I was averaging only 4 hours of solid sleep a night. Often, I'd end up taking a sleep aid and wake up with a groggy headache," she says.

The good news: Soon after upping her activity, she saw a huge, positive change in her sleep habits. While Schmidt still wakes up for a few minutes two or three times during the night, she no longer has trouble falling back to sleep.

"Now I walk almost daily, even if it's cold out. The yoga helps me relax and signals my body that it's bedtime. You hear myths that once you hit menopause, you'll never sleep well again, but exercise changed that for me."

So how does sweating help you snooze? "Exercise releases feel-good chemicals that boost your mood, which seems to reduce tension and anxiety that may interfere with your sleep," says Shawn Youngstedt, PhD, an associate professor in the department of exercise science at Arnold School of Public Health who has studied the exercise-sleep connection for nearly 20 years. "It also has a calming effect on the nervous system, which may increase the quality and duration of sleep."

Putting your body through a workout will also help ensure that you're physically tired by the time you crawl into bed. If you sat at a desk all day, pent-up energy could keep you tossing and turning.

THE FITNESS FIX FOR 40 WINKS

Ready to give our plan a try? We thought so. Follow the cardio recommendation on page 281, and aim to do a few minutes of restful yoga poses before you crawl into bed each night. (Find three great poses on page 280.) Need even more help? Turn to page 286 for more super simple tips to start sleeping more soundly tonight.

How We Conducted Our Research

How do we know our test panelists slept better? Because we couldn't sit in their rooms all night and watch them sleep—first, that would be creepy, and second, we have other things to do with our time—we outfitted them with a BodyMedia FIT Core Armband ($119; bodymedia.com). Worn around the upper arm, it monitors your activity level and calories burned throughout the day, as well as the amount of time you spend sleeping each night, minus any wakeful periods and bathroom visits.

For 1 week, the testers wore the armbands without changing their habits, allowing us to see how much they were moving and sleeping on a regular basis. Then we paired them with *Prevention*'s contributing editor and personal trainer, Chris Freytag, who asked them to incorporate at least 30 minutes of moderate to vigorous exercise into their day five or six times a week, as well as take a few minutes before bed to chill out with a few super-relaxing yoga poses.

To help them shed pounds faster, the group was asked to limit calories to around 1,600 a day. We also gave them a list of sleep hygiene tips from the National Sleep Foundation. (Find our list of science-backed, doze-inducing secrets on page 286.)

RELAX AND UNWIND WITH YOGA

The following three poses will help you prepare for slumber.

Legs-Up-the-Wall Pose

Sit on the floor with one side of your body grazing a wall. Swing your legs up against the wall and slowly lower your back and head to the floor, keeping your legs straight. Allow your hands to fall out to your sides, with your palms facing up. Breathe deeply, relaxing into the pose. Hold for 1 to 5 minutes.

Child's Pose

Kneel on a mat with your big toes touching and your knees spread mat-width apart. Lower your torso between your knees, bringing your forehead to rest on the mat and extending your arms. Breathe deeply, holding for up to 1 minute or even longer.

Happy Baby Pose

Lie on a mat and pull your knees to your chest. Place your hands on the outsides of your feet, opening your knees wider than your torso. Press your feet into your hands while pulling down on your feet, creating resistance. Breathe deeply, holding for up to 1 minute.

YOUR SWEAT Rx FOR RESTFUL NIGHTS

To reap the better-sleep benefits of exercise, aim to do 30 minutes of moderate to vigorous cardio at least 5 days a week.

"You need to work out hard enough that you get your heart pumping and break a sweat," says Freytag. "While brisk walks are simple and effective, find an activity you enjoy, whether that's taking a group cardio class at your local gym or a spin around the neighborhood on your bike."

And don't sweat it if the only time you have to sneak in a workout is a few hours before bedtime.

"The belief that evening exercise will keep you awake at night isn't true for the majority of people," says Dr. Youngstedt. However, if pre-sleep exercise does keep you awake, aim to fit it in at least 4 hours before bedtime.

Does 30 minutes sound daunting? Break it up into three 10-minute sessions throughout the day.

COUNTDOWN: 24 HOURS TO DREAMLAND

Follow our hour-by-hour plan to score some (seriously fabulous) z's.

Any bleary-eyed new mom or dad will tell you that the expression "sleep like a baby" is grossly misleading. Many babies sleep through the night only when they're put on a schedule. And you know what? If you can't remember the last time you got a good—and full—night's sleep, the same thing will work for you.

"Our bodies have an internal rhythm that takes cues from daytime behaviors, so the more strictly a person adheres to a schedule, the more his or her body will know when it's time to sleep," says Michael Breus, PhD, a clinical psychologist and the author of several books on sleep, including *The Sleep Doctor's Diet Plan: Lose Weight through Better Sleep*.

In today's world, where smartphones keep us tethered to work 24/7 and we all have more balls in the air than a Ringling Brothers clown, that might seem easier said than done. But there are plenty of good reasons to try, and not just because lack of sleep makes you crankier than a carb addict on Atkins. Research has linked sleep deprivation to some surprising conditions, including weight gain, reduced immunity, diabetes, and heart disease (not to mention that groggy "just give me another cup of coffee now" feeling that marks the days of the approximately one in four women who has trouble sleeping).

Find it hard to get yourself on any kind of schedule? We can help. We put together an hour-by-hour action plan that will help you fall asleep—and stay asleep—by 11 p.m. tonight. If your bedtime is earlier or later, adjust the times to compensate. Either way, you can look forward to finally getting the sleep you need.

7 a.m.: Wake up at the same time every day. It can be so tempting to sleep until noon on weekends, but 1 day of sleeping in can sabotage you for the rest of the week.

"Your internal biological clock craves consistency. The more you stick with one schedule, the easier it will be for you to fall asleep and wake up," says Dr. Breus. Ideally, you will go to bed around the same time every night so that you wake up at the same time in the morning. In fact, if you're getting enough sleep, experts say, you'll wake on your own a few minutes before your alarm goes off.

8 a.m.: Seek some light. When it's dark out, your body produces the hormone melatonin, which tells your brain it's time for sleep. Then daylight signals the body to suppress melatonin production so you can remain alert and awake. For a morning dose of alertness, get some direct sun exposure for 30 minutes within 1 hour of waking up. This is the time for taking your daily walk, sipping coffee on the back deck, or spending some quality time weeding the garden. Here's why: Being in the light helps reset your body's internal clock so it keeps you awake when you need to be and puts you to sleep at the right time.

"Light is the major cue that synchronizes our circadian rhythm, and getting enough exposure to it can solve many sleep problems," says Arthur Spielman, PhD, codirector of the Weill Cornell Center for Sleep Medicine at New York–Presbyterian Hospital.

If you can't get out in the morning or it's still dark when you wake up, ask your doctor if a commercially available light-therapy box that simulates natural sunlight might be right for you and, if so, which one she'd recommend. Dr. Breus suggests finding one that emits blue light with a wavelength around 450 nanometers that works faster than traditional light-therapy boxes.

2 p.m.: Drink your last latte. Caffeine can stay in your system for 8 or more hours, so try to avoid consuming any regular coffee, soda, or other highly caffeinated beverages too late in the day, says Judy Caplan, RD, the author of *GoBe-Full: Eight Keys to a Healthy Life* and a spokesperson for the Academy of Nutrition and Dietetics. If you're really sensitive to caffeine, you might also want to avoid or cut back on chocolate and tea, which contain smaller amounts of the stimulant. If you're ultrasensitive, even the smidge of caffeine in decaf could keep you up.

5:30 p.m.: Get in a workout. Good news for you gym rats: Working out is one of the best ways to ensure a good night's sleep.

"Exercise reduces the amount of time it takes to fall asleep and helps you sleep more soundly for longer periods," says Peter Walters, PhD, professor of applied health science at Wheaton College and the author of multiple studies about the link between sleep and exercise.

That doesn't mean you need to train for a triathlon. Exercising just 30 minutes 5 days a week can help you get some shut-eye. (For proof, consider the women who followed our program.) Schedule your workout for whenever you're most likely to stick with it, but if you find that late-night sweat sessions keep you awake, try to end it at least 4 hours before bedtime.

"During exercise, your body releases endorphins, and your heart rate increases," says Dr. Walters. "After you're finished, your heart and metabolism continue to function at an accelerated rate."

So if you're exercising close to bedtime, calm down by meditating or doing a few gentle yoga poses before you hit the sack.

6 p.m.: Limit fluids. If you're prone to waking in the middle of the night to use the bathroom, avoid drinking too much late in the day.

"Drink if you're thirsty, but otherwise don't guzzle fluids at night," says *Prevention* advisor Mary Jane Minkin, MD, clinical professor of obstetrics and gynecology at Yale University School of Medicine. "When you drink a beverage, it takes about 5 hours before your body filters it through the kidneys and into the bladder so you can urinate it out."

Get most of your eight daily glasses of water in before dinnertime.

6:30 p.m.: Eat a light meal. You've heard it before: Eat breakfast like a king, lunch like a prince, and dinner like a pauper. Well, that old saying isn't just a prescription for maintaining a healthy weight. It can also help you sleep better.

"Big, heavy meals take longer to digest, so if you lie down too quickly afterward, you're more likely to have acid reflux, which can interfere with your sleep," says Caplan.

Also, avoid spicy, acidic, and fried foods, which can cause indigestion and gastroesophageal reflux disease (GERD) in some people. If you're still hungry a

ANXIETY-PROOF BEDTIME

t's a common scenario: You have trouble falling asleep, and then you spend half the night worrying about the fact that you're still awake. The problem is, stressing about not sleeping will only make it a self-fulfilling prophecy.

"The harder you try to sleep and the more you think about it, the less likely it will happen," says Mary Susan Esther, MD, past president of the American Academy of Sleep Medicine.

The remedy: Get out of bed if you can't sleep. You want to associate the bed with sleeping, not worrying about not sleeping.

"People also believe that if they're having insomnia, they should spend more time in bed, but the exact opposite is true," says Gregg Jacobs, PhD, an insomnia specialist at the Sleep Disorders Center at the University of Massachusetts Medical School. "Reducing the amount of time in bed at night paradoxically doesn't reduce sleep time. It reduces awake time and increases sleep drive, which, in turn, makes the bed a stronger cue for sleep."

Ask your doctor about a form of cognitive behavioral therapy called restrictive sleep therapy.

"Sleep is a self-correcting process. If you reduce the amount of time you're allowed to sleep, it'll make you sleepier, you'll fall asleep quickly, and you'll gain the confidence that you can do so," says Arthur Spielman, MD, of Weill Cornell/New York–Presbyterian.

few hours after dinnertime, experts say it's okay to have a small bedtime snack, but choose wisely: Stick with 200 calories or less, and opt for snacks that contain complex carbs and a bit of protein, such as a small bowl of cereal with milk.

7 p.m.: Have your nightcap early. Sure, that glass of wine might make you drowsy and help you conk out, but it can also prevent you from falling into a deep sleep. In fact, a study by University of Michigan researchers found that women slept around 20 minutes less and woke more often throughout the night after consuming alcohol. No surprise: They also felt less rested.

"People fall asleep more easily with alcohol because it acts as a sedative, but once it wears off, it causes more arousals and sleep disruption later in the night," says Matt Bianchi, MD, PhD, director of the sleep division at Massachusetts General Hospital and assistant professor of neurology at Harvard Medical School. Bottom line: Stick with one or two alcoholic beverages—at most—around dinnertime, and cork the bottle 3 hours before bedtime.

8 p.m.: Prepare your room. "The bedroom is often the least carefully arranged room in people's houses," says William Dement, MD, PhD, past chief of the division of sleep at Stanford University and founder of the first sleep disorders clinic in the country.

To create a peaceful environment for sleeping, make sure there's no stress-inducing clutter and keep the room cool. (Around 65°F is optimal for most people.) Close room-darkening drapes or shades so no light peeks in to cut off melatonin production. If you're menopausal and prone to night sweats, keep an ice pack close by and dress lightly. No more flannels for you.

"These changes are simple, but many people don't make them," says Dr. Dement.

9 p.m.: Jot down your worries. Avoid that flood of predreamland jitters just as your head hits the pillow by designating a time earlier in the day to journal, write your to-do list, or work through any issues you've been mulling over.

"So many of my patients tell me they can't turn their brains off when they get in bed because it's their only time to be quiet and reflective all day long," says Mary Susan Esther, MD, past president of the American Academy of Sleep Medicine. With your worries and to-dos on paper, she says, "if your mind starts wandering when you're in bed, remind yourself that you've closed the book on the day, and there's nothing else you can do about the particular issue until tomorrow."

10 p.m.: Wind down. All that late-night Internet surfing you're doing before bed might be preventing you from falling asleep. A 2012 study from the Lighting Research Center found that a 2-hour exposure to light from self-luminous backlit devices such as tablets, e-readers, smartphones, and computers suppressed sleep-promoting melatonin by about 22 percent. Plus, texting or playing solitaire or Words with Friends can stimulate your brain so that you're too alert to fall asleep. Power down early.

"I give my patients an electronic curfew. An hour before bed, all devices

NATURAL SNOOZE INDUCERS

To drift off gently and naturally, try the following simple home remedies.

HOT BUBBLE BATHS: Taking a bath before bed relaxes your muscles and releases muscular tension, and it has a chemical effect as well. While you're in the tub, your core body temperature will rise, and then it will quickly drop when you get out. That decrease in temperature signals the brain to release melatonin, says sleep expert Michael Breus, PhD. The bubbles keep the water hotter longer.

MELATONIN: Some people say that taking these hormone supplements helps them sleep, but experts say it's not for everyone.

"Melatonin is a sleep regulator that affects your body's biological clock by signaling that it's time for sleep, but it doesn't make you feel sleepy," says Dr. Breus. "It's really for people who need to reset their clocks, such as shift workers or those dealing with jet lag."

Talk with your doctor about whether melatonin is right for you. If it is, take 1 milligram or less about 90 minutes before bedtime.

LAVENDER AROMATHERAPY: Some studies have shown that the scent of lavender acts as a mild sedative, helping you fall asleep faster and sleep more soundly. There are plenty of products to choose from, from massage oils and lotions to bath salts and reed diffusers.

must be turned off," says Dr. Breus. (One exception: If you find watching TV relaxing, some experts say that's okay, because it's not interactive.) After turning off your tech toys, keep the lights dim while you lay out your clothes for the next day and wash up for bed. Then do something soothing that clears your mind and relaxes your body, such as meditation (which some studies have suggested can increase melatonin production), reading, or doing some gentle full-body yoga stretches. (See page 280.)

11 p.m.: Lights out! Snuggle into bed and literally rest assured that you've planned the perfect day to help you get a good night's sleep.

LULLABIES: Nighttime lullabies don't just work on babies. Older people with sleep problems reported a 35 percent improvement after listening to 45 minutes of music before bedtime in a study in the *Journal of Advanced Nursing*. While the music doesn't have to be Brahms, we're not talking the Black Eyed Peas, 60 to 80 beats per minute is key, so seek out slow, steady music such as classical tunes or soft jazz.

VALERIAN ROOT: Multiple studies suggest that this herbal remedy might improve sleep quality without side effects. Valerian root seems to act as a sedative, reducing anxiety and calming the body before sleep. If you're going to give this alternative a try, take 400 to 900 milligrams of valerian extract between 30 minutes and 2 hours before bedtime for as many as 28 days, suggests the National Institutes of Health.

WHITE NOISE MACHINES: White noise machines block out background noise, such as a partner's loud snoring or street traffic, that might otherwise prevent shut-eye. Two worth trying are the HoMedics SoundSpa ($20; Bed Bath & Beyond) and the Brookstone Tranquil Moments Sleep Sound Therapy System ($130; brookstone.com).

AS GOOD AS GOLDIE

The perennially sunny actress shares her secrets for living well, aging well, cultivating spirituality, and raising happy, stress-resistant children.

Some people in this world have sunniness bequeathed to them as a birthright. Goldie Hawn has always seemed to be one of them. From the time we first fell for her in the movies *Cactus Flower*, for which she won the Oscar for best supporting actress, and *There's a Girl in My Soup*, Hawn has been one of those actresses who reflect light, from the top of her blonde mane (freakishly still natural, swears her hairstylist River Lloyd) to the tiny shimmering heart tattooed on her ankle.

Even the humor in her best roles is derived, ironically, from those moments when she is completely deflated, because it's so unexpected: The image of a wet, bedraggled Hawn on the poster for the movie *Private Benjamin* became a classic. Simply looking at her pout cracks us up.

Hawn would be the first to agree that she really was born with an abundance of natural optimism, though it's not present all the time and has always required practice. One of her favorite sayings is: "We are born with the seed of joy; it is up to us to nurture it."

Since the 1970s, Hawn, 68, has been a practitioner of meditation and living mindfully. Through the Hawn Foundation, she has brought the concept of mindfulness to 150,000 children around the world. Today, children in her MindUp program learn how they can reduce stress and anxiety by understanding where negative emotions live in the brain and taking charge of their own feelings. (She also released a book on the program, *Ten Mindful Minutes*.)

With a reclining Buddha watching over us, Hawn met with us in her glass-walled New York City penthouse. The living room is Indochined and feng shuied to the max; the furniture is all teak and pillows, the window treatments capped off with gold elephant heads. It was hard to resist plunking down and taking a nap on the opium bed that dominates the room. While Hawn got curled and fluffed for *Prevention*'s photo shoot, we discussed her secrets to looking great and feeling better.

Prevention: It seems these days that anyone and everyone who owns a yoga mat considers herself a Buddhist. We'd love to know what Buddhism means to you.

Hawn: Oh, I don't think of myself as a Buddhist. I was born Jewish, and I consider that my religion. But I've studied all religions, and as you learn more, you really learn that everyone's praying to the same God. I remember thinking about this once, being in Jerusalem, hearing the prayer calls of the Muslims, the church bells of the Christians, the Jews at the Western Wall [Hawn tears up]. It's not the idea of a particular religion that's important; it's the development of a spiritual life. Because spirituality creates well-being, health, and happiness. In Buddhism, it's called sangha—community. I believe having religion in your life creates the potential for long-lasting relationships.

> "Spirituality creates well-being, health, and happiness. In Buddhism, it's called sangha—community."

Prevention: And you should know. You've been with one partner (actor Kurt Russell) for nearly 30 years.

Hawn: Oh, yes. Yes. But anyway, it isn't what I think. It's what research has shown. I think what we're talking about with religion is connectivity.

Prevention: Yes, and you came quite early to meditation, at a time when it wasn't terribly mainstream. You were one of the first people talking about it.

Hawn: In the '70s, yes.

Prevention: And you've spoken about how you became a seeker at a time in your life when you were quite unhappy.

Hawn: Yes, I was anxious. Just when my fame was new. I was having what they call nonspecific panic attacks. I'd feel dizzy. My heart would start palpitating. I didn't like to be in crowds, because I'd get nauseous. You know, I had only wanted to be a dancer—that was my life. And next thing I knew, I was on this television series [the short-lived *Good Morning World*, right before she really gained fame as the body-painted go-go girl on *Rowan & Martin's Laugh-In*]. That hadn't been the plan. My dream was to go home and open a dancing school and get married and live a happy life. And moving in the world I was moving in, people were not what I would consider normal.

> *"If you learn how your brain functions, you can learn how to calm down and focus when you need to."*

I didn't want to be unhappy. I still remember sitting with my dad over a cup of coffee and saying, "Dad, I just want to be normal." And he said, "Go, you gotta get used to something: You're not normal."

Prevention: Smart dad.

Hawn: But I went to a psychologist because I had lost my smile. I was forcing an emotion that had been so natural to me and that now I didn't feel. I was out in space. I was no longer authentic. This happens to a lot of us at one time or another.

And so I spent many years in analysis, long after I lost that anxiety. Analysis is about self-discovery, and once you begin to answer questions about yourself, that's the beginning of one of the best parts of your life. But it was a gradual process.

Prevention: More recently, you've said you wanted to bring a form of self-knowledge to kids. After 9/11, you said you began thinking about the enormous amount of anxiety facing today's kids. So you assembled a team of researchers and created the program MindUp, with the premise that the more kids know about their own brains, the more they are able to regulate themselves and their behavior. Are you teaching them to meditate?

Hawn: We don't promote meditation in the class, but we do say, "Learn about your brain." And we do teach them to take "brain breaks." It's a science-based program. If you learn how your brain functions, you can learn to calm down and focus when you need to. So, for instance, if you're scared before a test, or your parents are breaking up, or whatever it is you fear, we help give them the ability to pay attention to the fear, to focus on their breathing, on the body's reactions. By tuning in to brain function, you can train the prefrontal cortex of the brain to make better choices.

I always remember this one little boy in one of our classrooms who I talked to about our program. He was 9. And I said to him, "So how does MindUp help you?" He says, "Well, the other day my best friend pushed me on the playground and really made me mad. But instead of hitting him back, I decided I'd just walk away and breathe and do a brain break. Because then I realized that I can't hit him back, because he won't be my best friend anymore." [Hawn smiles with delight.] Now, that's critical thinking! It's making good choices. It's quieting down your anger. But where do you make your good choices? This kid knew that you make them in the prefrontal cortex; that's the part of the brain that can manage and regulate emotion, that can analyze and retain information. [For more about meditation and mindfulness for us grownups, see page 293.]

Prevention: You have claimed that these methods help reduce the need to medicate kids who reportedly have attention deficit problems.

MEDITATION: TUNING OUT TO TUNE IN

Help, I can't shut off my brain! If this thought occurs to you more than now and again, meditation might offer not just peace but better health.

Here are Goldie Hawn's suggestions.

SHAKE HANDS WITH YOUR BRAIN. Hawn insists that if we know a bit about how the brain works, we can truly grasp why meditation is not just for those with a fondness for Birkenstocks and patchouli.

"Familiarize yourself with the parts of your brain and their function," Hawn says. "You will see that the benefits of meditation aren't just in your head. They're as physiological as the benefits of exercise on your muscles." For example, a 2011 study found that people who meditated 30 minutes a day for 8 weeks had increased gray matter in the hippocampus, an area critical to memory and learning, and a reduction of gray matter in the amygdala, a region associated with anxiety and stress. There were no changes in the brain matter of a control group that didn't perform mindfulness meditation.

DECIDE YOU WANT TO MEDITATE. Making something a priority for your well-being is half the battle. Take a little time to just sit and listen to your own breathing.

"It will probably be a bit irregular," Hawn says. Gradually, you'll learn to regulate your breathing and your brain.

GIVE YOURSELF AT LEAST THREE "BRAIN BREAKS" A DAY. Worried that meditating takes too much time? Research shows that meditating for 3 minutes 5 times a day is as beneficial to the body as doing it in a single 20-minute block of time.

Think of meditation not as something woo-woo but as an everyday task, like brushing your teeth. It's all about habituation, Hawn says—getting your brain and body used to the downtime. So do whatever it takes to establish a routine: Sit in a certain position, find a private spot in your home. The whole point of mindfulness meditation is to anchor your mind in the present and not allow it time to travel to the past and the future, which it does at lightning speed almost 24/7.

Hawn: Oh, I have seen it for myself. But I mean, there was a class [doing the MindUp program] in Vancouver that had some very challenged children. Some had been abused; some had seen genocide. Some of the parents were drug addicts. And do you know, half the kids in the class who were on medication for attention problems were able to go off it? There are kids who need medication, certainly, but the overmedicating of kids in our society is huge.

Prevention: Do you practice brain breaks with your grandsons? [Hawn's daughter, Kate Hudson, 34, recently gave birth to her second son, Bingham, and has a 9-year-old, Ryder. Hawn's son, Oliver, has two children, Wilder, 6, and Bodhi, 3.]

Hawn: **Yeah. They love it.**

Prevention: You look absolutely amazing. It's hard to believe you are a 68-year-old grandmother. You say that meditation and being mindful keeps you from holding on to anger. Has it also helped you deal with aging?

Hawn: No, no. What helps with aging is serious cognition—thinking and understanding. You have to truly grasp that everybody ages. Everybody dies. There is no turning back the clock. So the question in life becomes: What are you going to do while you're here?

Prevention: How about exercise and diet? You must be a fanatic.

Hawn: Not at all! I do try to do some form of exercise 4 days a week. At home in California, I'll bike up the mountain. Or I'll do Pilates or Spin. And I do eat a lot of greens. I eat healthily, but I'm not a vegetarian. I like to cook, and I tend to make those one-pot meat dishes of my Hungarian ancestors. Also, I make a great Bolognese. But you know what else is important? Just knowing how to play. Kurt and I get a lot of playtime in the home we built in Palm Desert.

Prevention: Your character Elise in *The First Wives Club* famously said, "There are three ages for women in Hollywood: babe, district attorney, and *Driving Miss Daisy*." Well, you haven't done any movies in about 10 years. Is that why?

Hawn: [Laughing] No, I don't think so. I just had such a need to concentrate on this one thing, on this foundation and on helping kids become better able to focus and organize their brains, to help them toward happiness. But now, well, recently I've been thinking about movies again. A lot. I'm beginning to miss that work.

Prevention: What do you miss most?

Hawn: **Making people laugh.**

Prevention: Will you go back?

Hawn: **Well, I like to say, "You never know what you don't know."**

"Everybody ages. Everybody dies. There is no turning back the clock. So the question in life becomes: What are you going to do while you're here?"

Part 6

BEAUTY
BREAKTHROUGHS

CHAPTER 27

BEAUTY FOODS

Eat your way to better skin. Enjoy the following 12 easy food fixes, and you'll have your most beautiful complexion ever.

The path to beautiful skin just might be through your stomach.

"When the body is out of balance, one of the first places it reveals itself is the skin," says Ruthie Harper, MD, a board-certified internist in Austin, Texas, who specializes in nutritional medicine. "If you're not getting the right nutrients, skin gets cheated out of what it needs for optimal health and beauty."

Learn to make the most of your body's skin/gastrointestinal (GI) connection with these 12 food fixes that give you a healthy, glowing complexion while warding off a host of skin conditions.

POWER UP WITH PROBIOTICS

When the stomach's natural flora gets out of whack because of stress, infection, or a course of antibiotics, you might experience digestive ills and skin problems such as acne, psoriasis, and eczema, as well as dullness and wrinkles.

"If your gut's bacteria balance is unfavorable, the toxic bacteria can leak through microscopic holes in the wall of your GI tract and travel throughout your body, including to your skin, causing inflammation that prevents the skin from functioning properly," says Frank Lipman, MD, an integrative physician and director of Eleven Eleven Wellness Center in New York City.

To prevent problems, keep your digestive tract populated with good bacteria, which "coat the lining of your gut and help seal it so unwanted substances can no longer leak out and cause irritation," says Whitney Bowe, MD, medical director of cosmetic and laser services at Advanced Dermatology in Ossining, New York.

Probiotics improve skin from the inside out, but applying them topically might also be beneficial.

"We have good and bad bacteria on our skin, just as we do in our gut," says Ellen Marmur, MD, an associate professor of dermatology and genetics at the Mount Sinai School of Medicine in New York City. "If the balance is off-kilter, it can result in acne or rosacea."

The right bacteria might also keep skin young.

"A study found that probiotics can stimulate skin's protective mechanism from the inside, and this may also happen with external application," cosmetic scientist Eric Perrier says.

How do you get the good bacteria? The best way is to take a probiotic supplement (available at most health food stores) or consume fermented foods such as kefir, yogurt, buttermilk, miso, kimchi, and sauerkraut. You should also eat foods that contain prebiotics, which are undigestible nutrients that stimulate the growth of good bacteria in your gut. Sources include whole grains, bananas, onions, and garlic.

SPRINKLE ON SUPER SEEDS

The healthy fats known as omega-3s are like manna from heaven for dry skin. They're anti-inflammatory, and they also moisturize skin so it stays soft and supple, and fine lines are less noticeable. Research shows that eating more omega-3–rich foods might even help protect against sun damage and skin can-

You might choose organic foods to eat, but what about organic products for your skin? If you want to buy organic in the beauty aisle, look for the NSF stamp. It's blue, with the letters NSF encircled and a leaf and the words "contains organic ingredients." This stamp indicates that the product is at least 70 percent organic and has passed guidelines set by health and environmental organization NSF International.

Items using the word organic that don't have this seal (or the USDA's familiar green-and-white organic stamp) might contain very few organic ingredients—or none at all.

cer. Salmon, sardines, and mackerel are omega-3 powerhouses. For people who prefer not to eat fish, flaxseed and chia seeds offer a great alternative.

"Just 1 ground tablespoon of these seeds has six times the recommended daily amount of omega-3s," Dr. Harper says. Try them sprinkled on salads, blended in smoothies, and as a crunchy topping for oatmeal.

PICK PURPLE PRODUCE

"The fatty acids in chia seeds keep skin soft."

Free radicals—molecules with unpaired electrons that are produced when skin is exposed to UV rays or environmental pollutants, such as carbon monoxide or cigarette smoke—set off a chain reaction that can damage virtually any molecule in the body, including the important cellular structures in the skin.

One of the best ways to neutralize free radicals is by eating foods that pack an antioxidant punch, such as berries, beans, and leafy greens. Purple, however, is the power color when it comes to your looks.

"Purple potatoes, purple cabbage, purple cauliflower, raspberries, and blueberries are all rich in anthocyanins, which is a type of antioxidant that also helps improve circulation," Dr. Harper says. "That increased blood flow helps bring skin the nutrients it needs to form new cells, collagen, and elastin."

SKIP THE SUGAR

More than your waistline suffers when you eat too much sweet stuff.

"Sugar is poison for the skin," Dr. Lipman says.

It is another cause of inflammation, and it also leads to glycation, which is a process that ages skin prematurely. Here's how: Sugar in your bloodstream binds to proteins and speeds the formation of advanced glycation end products (known as AGEs, coincidentally).

"AGEs stimulate enzymes in the skin that start chomping up collagen and elastic tissue," says Alan Dattner, MD, a holistic dermatologist in New York City.

The breakdown of collagen and elastin contributes directly to wrinkles, sagging, and uneven skin tone. No surprise, then, that a recent study in the *Journal of the American Aging Association* found that people with higher blood sugar levels were judged to look older than those with lower blood sugar.

If you can't curb your sweet tooth, eat slowly. That reduces glycation stress, which is a condition that damages skin. Also choose low-glycemic desserts to reduce the ill effects, suggest Japanese researchers who've studied the process.

Eliminating sugar—in all its forms—from your diet is the obvious, though somewhat extreme, solution. But even reducing your consumption by limiting it to the sugars contained in fruit, for example, can help, Dr. Dattner says.

How you consume sugar is also important to your glycemic level. Eating an Oreo a day for a week isn't as bad as polishing off an entire sleeve at once, because taking in large quantities of sugar at a time throws insulin levels out of whack.

COOK SOME CURRY

Perk up your meals with inflammation-fighting spices.

"Turmeric, also called curcumin, is a staple of many curries and helps reduce skin irritation, as do ginger and cinnamon," Dr. Harper says.

Some spices might also help protect you from sun damage. A recent study reported that turmeric supplementation (oral or topical) increases photo protection in skin. So add these skin-savvy spices to your diet.

"Turmeric and cinnamon reduce skin irritation."

EAT MORE FRUIT

First, an apple a day might keep the wrinkles away. Why? Because quercetin, which is an antioxidant in the peel of many varieties, provides hefty protection from the "burning" UVB rays that trigger skin cancer. A few of the apple varieties that offer the biggest dose are: Monroe, Cortland, and Golden Delicious. The next time you plan to spend time in the sun, pick one of them to start your day. (Of course, you still need to wear sunscreen.) Whatever variety you choose, be sure to eat the peel, which is the source of nearly all the antioxidants.

Another fruit to pick is strawberries. Just one cup has up to 130 percent of the Daily Value of vitamin C, which is a potent antioxidant that boosts production of collagen fibers that help keep skin smooth and firm. More C might mean fewer fine lines too. Women with lower intakes were likelier to have dry, wrinkled skin. Early research also shows that ellagic acid, which is an antioxidant abundant in strawberries, protects the elastic fibers that keep skin from sagging. Sweet!

GO FOR GREENS

In particular, eat more Romaine lettuce. Six leaves provide more than 100 percent of your Daily Value of vitamin A, which revitalizes skin by increasing cell turnover. The mineral potassium in Romaine "gives skin a refreshing boost of nutrients and oxygen by improving circulation," says Lisa Drayer, RD, author of *The Beauty Diet*.

As an extra health bonus: That same serving of Romaine contains 45 percent of the Daily Value of vitamin K, which a recent study shows activates a protein that supports vascular health—making a future with bulging leg veins less likely.

ORDER ITALIAN

Why? It's full of tomatoes. Eating tomatoes helps keep skin from turning red. Volunteers who consumed 5 tablespoons of high-in-lycopene tomato paste daily for 3 months had nearly 25 percent more protection against sunburn in one study. Even better, skin had more collagen, which prevents sagging. Another reason to toss an extra tomato into your salad: German scientists report that higher skin levels of this antioxidant correlate to fewer fine lines and furrows.

Even better: Research suggests that lycopene might also lower your chances of heart disease. In one study, women with the highest levels of it had a 34 percent reduced risk.

ENJOY SOME INCREDIBLE, EDIBLE EGGS

Lutein and zeaxanthin, two antioxidants found in eggs, more than quadrupled protection against the UV damage that leads to lines, brown spots, and cancer in one study on women. Skin was also markedly softer, firmer, and better hydrated.

As an added bonus: Eating just one egg a day significantly increases blood levels of lutein and zeaxanthin (but not cholesterol), which might stave off macular degeneration by protecting the retina from light damage, finds a study in the *Journal of Nutrition*.

TRY SOY

Fine wrinkles and skin firmness improved after women in their late thirties and early forties ate foods such as tempeh that contain the soy isoflavone known as aglycone, found one study. Volunteers consumed an amount of aglycone comparable to 3 ounces of tempeh a day for 12 weeks.

The best sources: whole foods. Try substituting edamame for any vegetable and tempeh or tofu for meat and poultry in stir-fries and soups.

GO NUTS

"Eating a handful of almonds every day boosts levels of vitamin E, one of the most important antioxidants for skin health," says Leslie Baumann, MD, a Miami Beach dermatologist. You'll get a surge in moisture too—a boon for those prone to dryness.

Another nut to enjoy is walnuts. These nuts are full of alpha-linolenic acid, an omega-3 fat that's a key component of the lubricating layer that keeps skin moist and supple. A $\frac{1}{2}$-ounce serving of walnuts provides 100 percent of the recommended daily intake of ALA.

Health bonus: Eating walnuts at dinner might deliver better shut-eye. Researchers at the University of Texas Health Science Center discovered that walnuts contain melatonin, a hormone that regulates sleep.

EAT MORE CHOCOLATE

We could probably stop there; who needs a reason? But women in one study positively glowed after drinking $\frac{1}{2}$ cup of cocoa made with dark chocolate, thanks to a significant increase in circulation that lasted 2 hours. But a daily cocoa habit might rejuvenate your complexion even more. Women who drank $\frac{1}{2}$ cup of cocoa high in flavonoids (as is dark chocolate) every day for 12 weeks in another study had significantly softer, smoother, and better hydrated skin. Try Nestle Hot Cocoa Dark Chocolate.

CHAPTER 28

THE NEW NATURALS

A fresh wave of alterna-treatments promises firmer, younger-looking skin. Do they really work?

If you always do what you've always done, you'll always get what you've always got. True in so many things. Here are some skin care treatments you probably haven't tried, in fact, maybe haven't even heard of. Are they worth giving a go?

THE TREATMENT: AYURVEDIC MEDICINE

What is it? This system of traditional Indian healing relies on techniques such as diet changes, breathing exercises, and botanical medicine to treat patients based on their dosha, or "body type."

Does it work? "The doshas seem to line up with skin types we're familiar with," says Jasmina Aganovic, an MIT–trained chemical and biological engineer and founder of the Stages of Beauty skin care line. "The Vata dosha typically coincides with dry skin; Pitta coincides with sensitive; and Kapha, with

"Grapeseed extract fights off skin-damaging free radicals even better than vitamins C and E."

oily or combination skin." Even so, there's no scientific evidence that treating your skin based on your dosha is beneficial, says Susan Stuart, MD, a dermatologist in San Diego.

However, there is proof that many of the plant-based ingredients used topically in Ayurvedic medicine can help you look younger. For example, "research shows that turmeric and ginger, both used frequently in Ayurvedic medicine, can reduce wrinkles," says Shyam Gupta, PhD, a chemist and founder of Bioderm Research, a cosmetic research company in Scottsdale, Arizona. And several studies show that grapeseed extract, another Ayurvedic ingredient, protects against photodamage.

The bottom line: It's okay to try products with Ayurvedic ingredients such as turmeric and ginger, but don't overhaul your beauty regimen based on your dosha just yet.

THE TREATMENT: ALKALINE DIET

What is it? A few studies have shown that acidity can be damaging to the body, so it's thought by some that eating mostly alkaline-forming (acid-lowering) foods such as fruits and vegetables might slow skin aging.

Does it work? There's no research proving this theory. (Our bodies do a good job of regulating acidity regardless of diet.) But there is anecdotal support. "My clients who eat 80 percent alkaline-forming foods notice fewer lines and

30-MINUTE WRINKLE REDUCER

Wrinkles are less noticeable after 30 minutes in a room with 70 percent relative humidity (RH) than in a room with 40 percent RH, reports a Japanese study. So flip on the humidifier before splurging on that pricey face cream.

more hydrated skin in weeks," says nutritionist Kimberly Snyder.

The bottom line: The diet won't erase wrinkles, but eating more fruits and veggies improves overall health, and that can only be good for skin.

THE TREATMENT: SKIN NEEDLING

What is it? In this painless procedure, you roll a needle-covered device over your face to create tiny, temporary pricks in your skin, which might trigger a healing response (similar to what occurs after a cut), leading to a smoother complexion.

Does it work? San Francisco dermatologist Kathy Fields, MD, who helped develop a home-needling device for Rodan + Fields, says her company's analysis shows using it can induce skin's collagen-building process and improve penetration of anti-aging ingredients applied afterward. But there aren't peer-reviewed studies of at-home devices, and Dr. Stuart believes needling is safer and more effective done in a dermatologist's office with a professional version of the tool.

The bottom line: When used before a retinol-based product, an at-home skin-needling tool can smooth skin, but it's likely that the retinol is doing most of the work.

THE TREATMENT: A CLEANSE

What is it? Some experts think that temporarily restricting your diet (whether with a cleanse, a juice fast, or a similar detox plan) can clarify your complexion and make your skin glow.

Does it work? "Most people's skin improves when they do a cleanse because they're removing foods that have a pro-inflammatory effect, and inflammation is the root of many skin issues, including rosacea, acne, and premature aging," says Frank Lipman, MD, an integrative physician and founder of Eleven Eleven Wellness in New York City.

"Most people's skin improves when they do a cleanse."

A cleanse won't turn back the clock, but eating less sugar and fewer starchy carbohydrates could be beneficial in the long run.

Although it's best to have an integrative medicine expert guide you in the cleansing process, it's possible to see benefits on your own. Dr. Lipman says avoiding caffeine, sugar, dairy, gluten, and meat for a few weeks can offer a short-term boost to your complexion. Research supports this theory to some extent. Gluten intolerances have been linked to skin issues for some people, and several studies have shown a correlation between dairy consumption and acne.

However, Mary Lupo, MD, a dermatologist and member of *Prevention*'s advisory board, says there are no studies showing that a temporary cleanse—no matter what types of food are restricted—can reduce cellular inflammation or provide any long-term skin benefits.

The bottom line: A cleanse won't turn back the clock, but eating less sugar and fewer starchy carbohydrates could be beneficial in the long run.

"These foods can spike blood glucose levels, and that accelerates aging of all organs, including the skin, says Dr. Lupo.

MASKS FROM MOTHER NATURE

Face masks might seem like an indulgence, but they offer extra rewards you can't get from your regular skin routine.

"Because the formulas remain on skin longer than other products you use, they have the ability to deliver more concentrated doses of beneficial ingredients," says Paul Jarrod Frank, MD, a dermatologist in New York City. The following three masks rely on nature's bounty to treat your skin issues.

MINERAL: Clairvoyant Beauty French Clay Mask with DMAE ($40; clairvoyantbeauty.com) draws out impurities, making pores look smaller.

VEGETABLE: The Body Shop Blue Corn Deep Cleansing Scrub Mask ($17; thebodyshop-usa.com) deep-cleans and exfoliates for softer skin.

FRUIT: ilike Organic Skin Care's Pumpkin & Orange Mask ($44; dermstore.com) moisturizes and brightens a dull, dry complexion.

NATURAL ALL-STARS

After reviewing ingredients, research company Organic Monitor named Intelligent Nutrients, John Masters Organics, and Aubrey Organics the top brands in the United States.

WASH THIS WAY. John Masters Organics Zinc & Sage Shampoo with Conditioner ($20; johnmasters.com) has a dozen certified organic ingredients—and no sulfates or synthetic fragrances.

SAVE YOUR SKIN. Aubrey Organics Rosa Mosqueta Night Creme ($23.50; aubreyorganics.com) staves off wrinkles with gentle anti-agers such as rosa mosqueta and primrose oil.

SMACK YOUR LIPS. Intelligent Nutrients Lip Delivery Antioxidant Gloss in Purple Maize ($24; intelligentnutrients.com) packs free-radical fighters from good-for-you superfoods such as acai berries and gets its pretty mauve color from purple corn.

CHAPTER 29

PREVENTION'S BEAUTY AWARDS

Celebrate—and elevate—your beauty with the following Prevention-*picked products. We tested dozens of products so you don't have to!*

It's been said that beauty is in the eye of the beholder, but *Prevention* believes that the only person with the power to decide what's pretty is you. Our goal isn't to promote one standard of beauty. Rather, we believe you should enhance what makes you unique with products that improve your skin and hair, imparting subtle changes that give you reason to celebrate—if only for a minute (privately!)—your beauty.

But where to start? With so many products available, how do you know which really work, are safe, and won't be irritating? Which ones will hydrate your skin, make your complexion smoother, or give you hair that's thicker, shinier, or softer? That's where *Prevention* comes in. The award winners presented here make you look great, and they also strengthen the health of your skin and hair. And that is definitely something to make a fuss over.

CLEAN SWEEP

Get your skin in shape with these six complexion perfecters, chosen with the help of our judging panel: 275 readers, 10 dermatologists and chemists, and an independent lab.

Every woman wants to look like herself, only a little bit better. In fact, more than half of American women say they strive to appear "refreshed," while just 4 percent want to look "like a movie star," according to a recent survey from Harris Interactive. That's why we know you'll love these skin-healing products that make it easy for you to look your best.

"My skin felt softer immediately," one tester raved.

Best Cleanser/Cleansing System

Clarisonic Mia 2 Sonic Skin Cleansing System ($149; clarisonic.com)

You know how great your teeth feel after a cleaning at the dentist's office? Washing daily with this face brush and its accompanying cleanser gives your face the same instant gleam. The soft exfoliating bristles oscillate at sonic-level speed, clearing dirt and dead skin cells so that the moisturizers and anti-agers you use afterward will be more effective.

"This cleansing system reduced the amount of blemish-causing bacteria on testers' skin up to 22 percent, and those who used it ended up with less redness and fewer wrinkles and UV spots over time," says judge Marina Peredo, MD, associate clinical professor at Mount Sinai School of Medicine. Expect the brush head to last 3 to 4 months. Two replacement heads cost $40.

Best Day Moisturizer

Philosophy Miracle Worker SPF 55 Miraculous Anti-Aging Fluid ($57; philosophy.com)

"This formula is the most hydrating one we tested—great for temporarily plumping fine lines," says judge Jennifer Linder, MD, assistant clinical professor at UC–San Francisco.

For long-term improvements such as less redness and fewer spots, the lotion also features collagen-stimulating peptides, calming chamomile and aloe, and antioxidants from spruce-wood extract that all help boost the efficacy of the high SPF.

Best Night Cream/Serum

Neutrogena Rapid Wrinkle Repair Serum ($22; drugstores)

This lightweight serum fights aging like a heavyweight, and it beat out finalists that cost almost five times as much! The gentle retinol complex left testers' skin with up to 15 percent fewer fine lines and a 15 percent smoother texture after 6 weeks.

"Typically, retinol can dry skin when you first start using it," says judge Mary Lupo, MD, clinical professor at Tulane Medical School and a *Prevention* advisor. "But this formula of retinol with hyaluronic acid and glucose makes it work fast with few side effects."

"This works quickly, and results last longer than other products," a tester said.

Best Facial-Hair Remover

Olay Smooth Finish Facial Hair Removal Duo ($25; drugstores)

Women with a whisper of whiskers know it can be time-consuming and irritating to keep upper lips, chins, and cheeks fuzz-free, but this depilatory duo makes the chore easier. Its skin-guarding balm (step 1) "contains fatty acids and vegetable-derived conditioners that help protect skin," Dr. Linder says. The depilatory cream (step 2) "is infused with chamomile and aloe that further tone down irritation."

Testers said the formula was gentle (no telltale red upper lip), smelled "pleasant, not chemical," and offered results that lasted well over a week—longer than any of the other finalists.

Best Repair Treatment

RoC Retinol Correxion Max Wrinkle Resurfacing System ($27; drugstores)

Even the most effective moisturizer can't do everything, so it makes sense to supplement your regimen with a booster that treats imperfections such as redness caused by aging, spots, and stubborn lines. Every tester who used this system saw overall redness decrease and ended up with, on average, 10 percent fewer wrinkles. (One reader had 27 percent fewer!)

"The first step, a lotion, has retinol, which rejuvenates aging, damaged skin," says judge Marguerite Germain, MD, a dermatologist in Charleston, South Carolina. "The second step, a serum, has a special zinc-and-copper complex that interacts with the first product to generate a safe and undetectable microcurrent, designed to drive the ingredients deeper into skin."

Testers used the system nightly for 6 weeks, but those with sensitive complexions (such as one of our testers, who found it too potent) can use it just two or three times a week and still see similar benefits, Dr. Germain says.

Best Eye Cream

Lancome Renergie Eye Multiple Action ($78; lancome-usa.com)

All the lucky women who tried this rich eye cream were hooked. It moisturizes, and it also softens wrinkles: Visia pictures taken by our dermatologist judge showed one tester's crow's-feet were reduced by 32 percent after 6 weeks.

"The jojoba butter hydrates, so lines are immediately less noticeable, and yeast and bean extracts help create younger, fresher cells in the long run," says Dr. Peredo.

A clever bonus: The lid opens to reveal a concealer with SPF 15 (available in three shades) that hides discoloration.

COLOR YOURSELF HEALTHY

The following eight products—chosen as winners by our panel of 275 readers, 10 dermatologists and chemists, and an independent lab—improve the condition of your skin, your lips, and even your lashes every time you use them.

Best Blush

VMV Hypoallergenics Skin Bloom Blush (available in eight shades; $40; vmvhypoallergenics.com)

Cheeks are typically the driest area of your face, and the pigments in many blushes can dehydrate them further, according to judge Ni'Kita Wilson, chemist and VP of research and innovation at Englewood Lab. That's a nonissue with this formula's addition of moisturizing virgin coconut oil. Some other factors that make the powder better than basic blush: no parabens, no fragrance, no phthalates, and (in four of the shades) no synthetic dyes.

"For people with an allergy to any of those ingredients, this blush would be a good option," says judge Ranella Hirsch, MD, assistant clinical professor at Boston University School of Medicine.

Beyond the makeup's health advantages, our testers were excited about how great it made them look—and how others noticed too.

"I got a compliment on my 'natural glow' and another on the pretty color of my cheeks the day I wore this," one said.

Best Lip Color

Bite Beauty Lush Lip Tint (available in six shades; $24; sephora.com)

With every swipe of this lipstick, the creamy B running through the center of the bullet delivers a dose of resveratrol.

"It's an antioxidant that can have a protective effect when applied topically," Dr. Hirsch says. If you ingest some of the color (it happens naturally as you lick your lips or talk), no worries. It doesn't contain synthetic dyes, fragrances, parabens, or petrochemicals. What testers liked best, however, were the long-lasting colors and soft texture.

"I didn't feel like I was wearing lipstick," one said. "It goes on smooth and light," another said.

"After a drink, the color stayed on my lips, not on the cup," said a third. "It's like a lip balm," Dr. Hirsch notes.

Best Foundation

Clinique Repairwear Laser Focus All-Smooth Makeup SPF 15 (available in 12 shades; $32.50; clinique.com)

The more you wear this foundation, the less of it you need. The moisturizing formula evens out skin tone and hides redness. One tester called the coverage "just right—not too light, not too heavy". Vitamin E and sunscreen protect against damage and discoloration, while a peptide and a botanical extract

PRETTY SIMPLE

Makeup artist Sonia Kashuk explains here how to look your best in just four simple steps.

LIP AND CHEEK TINT: "Brighten your complexion by blending the same rosy shade on your lips and the apples of your cheeks," suggests Sonia. Try 100% Pure Fruit Pigmented Lip and Cheek Tint ($15; 100percentpure.com).

CLEAR BALM: This multitasker adds shine to lips, but "you can also use it to tame errant brow hairs or even to moisturize your cuticles," notes Sonia. Try Vaseline Lip Therapy ($1; Walmart).

SHEER FOUNDATION: Even out your skin by smoothing on a lightweight foundation, such as Sonia Kashuk Perfecting Luminous Foundation ($10.50; Target). It can also double as concealer: "Use a gentle tapping motion with your ring finger to apply a slightly thicker layer on areas where you need extra coverage," Sonia says.

BLACK MASCARA: "No look is complete without mascara," says Sonia. Pick a tiny tube, such as Sally Girl Mini Mascara ($1; Sally Beauty). This forces you to replace it every 3 months, which is smart, considering that one study showed that 36 percent of regular-size mascara tubes are contaminated with bacteria by that time.

(*Siegesbeckia orientalis*, a Southeast Asian herb) help provide a better support system to plump up and fill in lines.

"On average, testers using this for 6 weeks had a 10 percent improvement in their skin tone and texture," says judge Jeanine Downie, MD, a dermatologist in Montclair, New Jersey.

"This covered all my dark spots really well. Impressive," raved a tester.

Best Concealer

Clinique Even Better Concealer (available in 12 shades; $19.50; clinique.com)

With 43 new foundations and 30 new concealers entered in our awards, we were impressed when the same brand came out on top in both categories. Testers liked how well this cover-up blended and its ability to work on all types of imperfections. One who used it under her eyes said it made her look "refreshed and more awake," while another praised its ability to hide "spots and the redness around my nose."

Dr. Hirsch says that the formula has vitamin C, typically used in skin creams to help fade discoloration. Although our testers didn't have measurable improvements on that front, Dr. Hirsch's thinking is: "Between a regular concealer and one with vitamin C, it's worth trying the vitamin C one."

"It lasted all day and didn't cause dryness under my eyes," a tester said.

Best Eye Makeup

Bare Escentuals BareMinerals Ready Eyeshadow 2.0 (available in 22 shade duos; $20; bareminerals.com)

This solid powder shadow offers the benefits of mineral makeup—pigments derived from natural sources, a formula that's excellent for sensitive skin—as well as amazing color payoff (one swipe delivers the hue you see in the pan). On top of that, it's formulated with anti-inflammatory caffeine, soothing cucumber, and cold-pressed borage oil.

"Borage oil is a great moisturizing skin conditioner, and it may contribute to this shadow going on so smoothly, with an almost-gel-like consistency," Dr. Hirsch says. One tester with blepharitis (a common condition that causes sensitivity and inflammation around the eyes) said most shadows irritate her eyes, but this one didn't, and she "absolutely loved" it. Another tester with "very oily eyelids" was impressed that the color "lasted for hours without creasing."

Best Mascara

Rimmel London Volume Accelerator Mascara (available in two shades; $9; drugstores)

They lengthen, thicken, and darken. But how many mascaras can actually prevent age-related lash thinning? This formula does, thanks to Procapil. Although it's not a drug like the ingredient in the prescription lash-growth product Latisse, Procapil "was designed to counteract alopecia [hair loss], and data shows it can help prevent lash loss without side effects," Wilson says.

Does it make lashes grow longer? Not exactly, but the formula also has caffeine, which might stimulate the hair follicle to become more active. Testers who tried it were blown away by the results.

"Using this instead of regular mascara was like driving a luxury car after being behind the wheel of a basic middle-of-the-road sedan for so long," one said.

"The mascara highlighted my thin lashes without clumps," another tester said.

Best Primer

Olay Regenerist Wrinkle Revolution Complex ($25; drugstores)

Ten years ago, primer was something you put on a wall. But a pre-makeup potion has quickly become part of many women's routines because it makes skin look smoother and helps cosmetics last longer.

This winning version goes even further. Its blend of moisturizers and micro-fillers makes pores and lines less noticeable on contact, while "peptides repair collagen, and niacinamide, an antioxidant, helps treat hyperpigmentation and inflammation," says judge Heidi Waldorf, MD, associate clinical professor at Mount Sinai School of Medicine. "The vertical line between my brows improved after a few weeks of using this," one tester reported.

Best Makeup Remover

La Fresh Eco-Beauty Waterproof Makeup Remover (24 wipes for $10; lafreshgroup.com)

Dermatologists tell us to take off our makeup at the end of the day, but some removers can be irritating, and anything with abrasives or particulates can't be used near eyes. These gentle wipes got the thumbs-up from judges because they're soaked with a safe-on-eyes solution that has olive, jojoba, grapeseed, and sesame oils to leave skin moisturized. Testers were fans of the "easy and convenient" way the wipes whisked away even waterproof eye makeup in a stroke or two.

"I have very sensitive skin, and these don't sting at all," one said.

"The remover wipes conditioned the skin around my eyes," reported another.

HAVE A GOOD HAIR DAY—EVERY DAY

There's a big difference between your products and these strand savers, chosen by our panel of 275 readers, 10 doctors and chemists, and an independent lab, and that's not just splitting hairs.

Best Hairspray

L'Oreal Paris EverStyle Strong Hold Styling Spray ($7; drugstores)

This spray got the highest marks of all the stylers we evaluated. Testers raved that the formula, which contains moisturizing glycerin and orange-peel oil, "wasn't sticky" and "held all day with one application." And it did so without alcohol, which "can strip hair of its natural sebum, leading to damage," judge Ni'Kita Wilson says.

"It made my hairstyle last all day through rain and humidity," said one tester.

Best Shampoo

Burt's Bees Super Shiny Mango Shampoo ($8; drugstores)

Suds remove dirt, but they also remove your hair's natural layer of protective sebum, leaving strands more prone to breaking. But hair washed with this low-sudsing shampoo had 32 percent less breakage than untreated hair after being stroked 10,000 times by a mechanized brush, according to our laboratory tests.

"The formula is also sulfate free, which means the cleansing agents are gentler," judge Arun Nandagiri, cosmetic chemist and founder of Bria Research Labs in Libertyville, IL says. "That bodes well for color-treated hair too, because the pigment is less likely to wash out."

Judge Marguerite Germain, MD, adds that using the shampoo makes your scalp healthier, thanks to "thyme oil, which has antioxidants, and mango-seed oil, a moisturizer."

Best Conditioner

Clear Scalp & Hair Therapy Strong Lengths Nourishing Daily Conditioner ($6; drugstores)

It's common for a woman's hair to thin as she gets older, which is why it's big news that using a conditioner such as this one can actually thicken hair.

"It has zinc pyrithione, which has been scientifically proved to promote and sustain increased hair growth," Dr. Germain says. "And its conditioning ingredients, such as sunflower-seed oil, bulk up strands and protect them, so they can grow longer."

Nandagiri says it's formulated to cling to the most damaged spots on your strands, which leads to shinier, smoother hair over time. How much smoother? Our lab tests showed that hair treated with the product was four to five times easier to comb than untreated hair.

"Panthenol in this conditioner promotes healthy hair growth," said judge Marguerite Germain, MD.

NATURAL SUPPLEMENTS FOR HEALTHY HAIR

Can a supplement really help your hair grow? We asked Jennifer Peterson, MD, a dermatologist in Houston, to weigh in on pills that promise thicker hair.

FEMBODY NUTRITION HAIR, NAILS & SKIN BEAUTY ACTIVATOR: A dose has 3,000 micrograms of biotin, a vitamin shown to improve nail thickness, which is often correlated with thicker hair. "Dermatologists have recommended biotin to patients with thin hair for decades," says Dr. Peterson. ($25; GNC)

NUHAIR DHT BLOCKER: Hair loss in men is often due to the influence of high levels of the hormone DHT, but an herb or supplement claiming to inhibit DHT probably won't benefit women. NuHair's Hair Regrowth Tablets for Women with biotin are more likely to help. ($26; nuhairproducts.com)

VIVISCAL EXTRA STRENGTH: This slowed rate of hair loss after 2 months and increased hair count after 6 months in a non-placebo-controlled study funded by the company. "Researchers think the marine extracts and silica in the pills may be responsible for improvements," says Dr. Peterson. ($50; viviscal.com) ess is better when it comes to the chemicals in hair dye. That's why we like Tints of Nature Permanent Colour ($18; Whole Foods). It covers gray but uses low levels of peroxide and phenylenediamine—ingredients that can dry hair and irritate the scalp—and contains no ammonia, which can wear away the cuticle that keeps hair shiny and holds in color molecules.

Best At-Home Hair Color

Couture Colour LuxeBlend Creme Hair Colour ($30; couturecolour.com)

Hair dye can cover grays, flatter your skin tone, and plump strand volume, but it can fade in as few as five shampoos and typically contains ammonia, which can be drying. Lab tests showed hair dyed with this at-home kit had 45 percent less color loss than hair dyed with others we tested. Plus, unlike the others, it's ammonia free.

A dose of pequi fruit oil in the dye and after-treatment might be the reason the color lasts, according to Wilson. "The ingredient coats hair to lock in color molecules," she says. "This dye's antioxidants enhance color vibrancy."

Best Volumizing Styler

Dove Style+Care Nourishing Amplifier Mousse ($4; drugstores)

Testers couldn't stop gushing about this mousse: "I live in a really humid area, and this gave my hair more volume and bounce without making it frizzy or limp," one said.

Wilson says that the mousse's fluffy texture lifts hair, while polymers in the formula wrap around individual strands to make them appear thicker and protect them from damage. "It also contains two conditioning agents that make hair soft, not crunchy, and easy to brush out at the end of the day," she says.

"The volume from this mousse lasted through a day of chasing after the kids!" one tester said.

Best Smoothing Styler

Nexxus ProMend Split End Binding Smoothing Shine Serum ($12; nexxus.com for retailers)

How did this serum outshine its competition? By calming frizz and repairing damage at the same time. It seals together 86 percent of split ends through a formula that contains "a positively charged polymer that wraps around the frayed tips and a negatively charged polymer that attaches itself on top, fusing the ends with a protective shield," Wilson says.

Testers gave it praise for smoothing unruliness without weighing down strands. "It was so lightweight, like I had nothing on my hair," one said.

BONUS! LOVE THE HAIR YOU HAVE

The only constant in life is change, and that goes for your hair too. Learn how your strands transform with age, and then use our quiz and guide to get your best hair ever.

You probably have a mental picture of yourself that's been in place for years: "I'm the short brunette with the curly hair," for example. But at some point, what's actually on your head no longer matches the image you carry in your head. "Most people know that hair color changes, but not many realize that texture does too," says Heather Woolery-Lloyd, MD, a dermatologist in Miami.

"Recent research shows that individual fiber thickness, or diameter, actually increases in your early thirties before peaking and declining from the late thirties or early forties and onward," says Pantene principal scientist Jeni Thomas, PhD. Density—the number of strands on your head—also changes. And then there's the wild card: curvature.

"Studies suggest that fiber shape and curvature become more irregular with age," Dr. Thomas says. For example, a woman with uniform ringlets in her thirties may end up with half-wavy, half-kinky curls in her sixties.

To ensure your current styling strategies match the strands you have today, find your hair type and learn to make the most of it with the quiz and guide that follow.

Quiz: What's Your Hair Type?

1. **DIAMETER:** Give yourself a diameter score of 1 to 5, with 1 being incredibly fine. Need help? Pluck a strand and roll it between your index finger and thumb. If you can't feel it at all, give yourself a 1. If it feels like a piece of thread, give yourself a 5.

Diameter score: _____

2. **DENSITY:** Give yourself a density score of 1 to 5, with 1 being sparse. If you can see your scalp between hairs and the base of your ponytail is smaller than a dime, you're a 1. If your scalp isn't visible and you shed a lot but your hair doesn't get thinner, give yourself a 5.

Density score: _____

3. **CURVATURE:** Comparing your hair with other women's, give yourself a curvature score of 1 to 5, with 1 being extremely straight (straighter than most other women's) and 5 being extremely curly (curlier than most). If your hair is wavy when you air-dry, you're a 3.

Curvature score: _____

Add the three numbers for your total score: _____

3 to 6: Fine Hair

Wash: Use a noncreamy shampoo, such as Redken Body Full Shampoo ($14.50; redken.com); transparent formulas are less likely to weigh down hair. Follow with a light conditioner. Aveda Invati Thickening Conditioner ($25; aveda.com) has ginseng to improve scalp circulation, so hair gets the nutrients necessary for growth.

Style: Apply a heat-activated mousse, such as Suave Professionals Volumizing Mousse ($3; drugstores). Then blow-dry, using a round brush to build volume if your hair is straight or a diffuser to prevent frizz if you have curls.

"Heat-activated products are like the starch you use on a shirt before ironing. They give the fabric—or in this case, hair—structure," says Dove celebrity stylist Mark Townsend. And consider coloring your hair, because dyes, such as Garnier Nutrisse Nourishing Color Foam ($9; drugstores), bulk up strands so they appear thicker.

Your best cut: Fine hair tends to look flat and limp if it gets long, so keep it shoulder length or shorter.

"The goal is not to overlayer your hair, because that can make it look thinner," says Yvette Gonzalez, senior stylist at Sahag Workshop in New York City.

7 to 11: Normal Hair

Wash: All hair can become drier with age, so you should wash less frequently than you did in your twenties. A shampoo with natural hydrators such as argan oil adds shine without causing buildup. Try Nexxus Frizz Defy Frizz Protection Shampoo ($10; drugstores). Next, use a smoothing conditioner. Pantene AgeDefy Conditioner ($8; drugstores) controls unruly grays without weighing hair down. Stop rinsing before the ends feel squeaky clean.

"A little conditioner left behind acts like a moisturizing treatment and helps prevent frizz," says Suave Professionals stylist Jenny Cho.

Style: Frizz is the most common complaint for this hair type, says New York City stylist Eva Scrivo. When humidity is in the air, it gets drawn into strands, causing the cuticle to expand and creating frizz, Scrivo says. Because hair that's already hydrated draws less water from the air, there's less frizz. So bring on the moisture and skip gels or sprays that list dehydrating alcohol as an ingredient. Go for a smoothing serum or styling cream instead. If you have straight or wavy hair, John Frieda Frizz-Ease Sheer Solution ($10; drugstores) is a great option. For curls, choose something a little richer, such as Yes To Carrots Anti-Frizz Serum ($8; drugstores) with hydrating mango seed butter.

Your best cut: Let your stylist see your hair in its air-dried state, so she can work with the natural curvature.

"Even if you plan to alter your texture with styling—by straightening it with a brush, for example—a cut that suits your hair in its natural condition will be most flattering," stylist Mark Townsend says.

12 to 15: Thick Hair

Wash: Thick or coarse hair needs extra moisture to remain smooth and shiny. The best shampoos for your hair type contain rich, hydrating ingredients. They often give shampoo an opaque, pearly quality that makes it look almost like conditioner. Try L'Oreal Paris EverCreme Cleansing Conditioner ($7; drugstores), which is a low-lather formula that cleans hair without high-foaming surfactants that can remove moisture. As for conditioner, the thicker your hair, the thicker your conditioner should be. Try one with a pudding-like consistency, such as Matrix Biolage Exquisite Oil Conditioner with Moringa Oil ($18; matrix.com). No matter which conditioner you choose, "leave it on at least 3 minutes before rinsing so your hair soaks up all the smoothing ingredients," says Glyn Roberts, a scientist in the research and development department at Nexxus.

Style: Your thick hair can probably support a style without mousse, gel, or hair spray. What you need instead are products that smooth unruliness and tame bulkiness, such as smoothing creams, oils, and balms. Try Garnier Fructis Sleek & Shine Moroccan Sleek Oil Treatment ($6; drugstores), which works well on straight or wavy strands, or Intelligent Nutrients Certified Organic Styling Pomade ($29; intelligent nutrients.com), a great option for curls and textured hair.

Your best cut: The right layering technique will help keep your hair from forming a pyramid. Stylist Eva Scrivo suggests triangular layers: "They balance thick hair's natural tendency to take on a pyramid shape by creating the opposite shape, an upside-down pyramid, or a triangle."

6"–10" THE DISTANCE TO HOLD HAIR SPRAY FROM HAIR SO PROPELLANTS DISSIPATE, ALLOWING ONLY THE STYLING INGREDIENTS TO REACH STRANDS, SAYS AQUAGE COFOUNDER LUIS ALVAREZ.

GET YOUR BODY BEAUTIFUL

Here are the best products for protecting and perfecting the skin below your chin, as judged by 275 readers, 10 experts, and one independent testing lab.

Best Body Wash

SheaMoisture Olive & Green Tea Body Wash ($10; Walgreens)

This all-natural cleanser took top honors in part because of what it doesn't contain: Its rich, creamy lather comes from coconut oil and a sugar-beet derivative instead of sulfates, which can be irritating and drying.

Judge Joel Schlessinger, MD, past president of the American Society of Cosmetic Dermatology and Aesthetic Surgery and founder of lovelyskin.com, was also impressed that the formula has no skin-irritating synthetic fragrances—something our testers, who raved about the light honeysuckle scent, were excited to learn. But in the end, the addition of skin-boosting ingredients gave this body wash the win.

"The green tea extract helps protect skin from damage and also has an anti-inflammatory effect," Dr. Schlessinger says. Plus, the formula contains avocado oil, which is rich in vitamins and minerals that help moisturize and regenerate skin cells.

"Green tea extract helps protect skin from damage," one tester said.

Best Body-Hair Remover

Schick Hydro Silk Razor ($10; drugstores)

All razors remove hair, but this slick-looking instrument actually improves the condition of your skin in the process. The blades are surrounded by a slim head coated with a water-activated moisturizing serum.

"As you shave, the serum delivers proteins, vitamins, and shea butter to rejuvenate skin," says judge David Bank, MD, assistant professor at Columbia University/NY–Presbyterian Hospital says. Multiple testers noted how the moisturizers made for a cleaner shave, but they also liked the easy-to-grip handle and the way the head maneuvered over tricky spots such as knees and ankles.

"The water-activated serum moisturizes," said a tester.

Best Self-Tanner

Dr. Dennis Gross Alpha Beta Glow Pad for Body with Active Vitamin D ($45; sephora.com)

It's hard to develop self-tanners that do more than tint skin, explains judge Wilson. But this formula also "speeds cell renewal and kick-starts collagen production," Dr. Bank says. More important, it created the best bronze our testers had ever gotten sans sun—without the funky faux-tanner smell.

Best Sunscreen

L'Oreal Paris Sublime Sun Hydra Lotion Spray SPF 50+ ($11; drugstores)

Every dermatologist will tell you that sunscreen is the best anti-aging product. So what makes this one the best of the best? In addition to blocking UVA and UVB rays with a blend of photostabilized (won't deteriorate with exposure to UV light) sunscreens, it has "vitamin E and white grapeseed extract, which work together to protect against free radicals and keep skin healthy and youthful looking," says Dr. Bank.

Our testers also liked how the continuous spray allowed for one-handed application, and they preferred the lotion-formula mist to clear mists, because it left skin moisturized without feeling sticky, and they could see where they were applying it.

Best Body Lotion

Aveeno Positively Ageless Skin Strengthening Body Cream ($10; drugstores)

This lotion promises to improve the texture and elasticity of skin, and Dr. Schlessinger was able to prove it does just that. "The before-and-after photographs we took clearly showed better skin texture and tone," he says.

What magic ingredient was responsible? He hypothesizes that it's moisturizing glycerin, but there's also a cocktail of botanicals—including extracts of algae, mushroom, and flowering southernwood, a variety of sagebrush—with antioxidant qualities that can help protect skin from both damage and dehydration.

Testers' favorite benefit was the fact that, over time, skin felt softer even on days they didn't use it.

Best Hand Cream

Philosophy Hands of Hope Hand and Cuticle Cream ($18; philosophy.com)

This rich cream wowed, hands down. Testers were fascinated by images showing how much better the backs of their hands looked after using it for 6 weeks.

"We noted enhancements in roughness, scaling, and even brown spots," Dr. Schlessinger says.

But several creams offered similar perks. So why did this one stand out? According to the testers, it was the only one that hydrated without making hands either slippery or smelly. One tester's husband liked the simple tube and unscented formula so much, he started using it too.

HOW WE PICKED THE WINNERS

To select the winning products, a panel of judges reviewed more than 1,700 products launched from April 2011 to June 2012 and chose 130 finalists. Each finalist was tested with criteria appropriate to its category.

Body lotions, face creams, and foundations were used by readers for 6 weeks under the supervision of a dermatologist, who determined winners using tools such as the Visia Complexion Analyzer by Canfield.

The top shampoos, conditioners, and hair dyes were tested at an independent lab under the supervision of a cosmetic chemist, while the hairstyling products were tested for 6 weeks by readers who filled out evaluation forms that were reviewed by experts.

Products such as self-tanners were tested by an independent lab and/or readers. For more details, and to check out the runners-up and get a behind-the-scenes look at testing, visit prevention.com/celebrate.

THE SURPRISING SECRET
TO BETTER-LOOKING SKIN

As teens, we obsessed over keeping pores squeaky clean. Now we have another reason to keep tabs on them.

"Pores look stretched around the edges when collagen breaks down and skin starts to sag," says Jennifer Linder, MD, a dermatologist and the chief scientific officer at PCA Skin. While we can't change pores' size, we can preserve protective collagen and keep oil at bay by adopting these tips from Dr. Linder.

PROTECT THEM. Sun exposure breaks down collagen, prompting pores to sag and appear larger, so as always, slather on SPF 30 daily. At night, consider a cream or serum with vitamin C and retinol to increase collagen and keep pores tight. Neutrogena Rapid Tone Repair Moisturizer SPF 30 has it all ($21; drugstores).

MINIMIZE THEM. Make pores less noticeable by using a pore-tightening alpha-hydroxy acid astringent toner daily and a clay-based oil-absorbing mask weekly. We like Dermalogica Skin Refining Masque ($40; dermalogica.com). For stronger results, see your dermatologist for a salicylic acid peel ($50 to $200), which will clear away excess oil and strengthen follicle walls.

CAMOUFLAGE THEM. Makeup with mica, a mineral that sops up oil, minimizing pores, and boron nitride, which refracts light, can make pores less obvious. BareMinerals Ready Foundation Broad Spectrum SPF 20 ($29; bareminerals.com) includes both.

CHAPTER 30

COLOR THERAPY

Somewhere in the rainbow, dreams that you dare to dream—of younger skin, shinier hair, and brighter eyes—really do come true!

It probably won't surprise you that color has a tremendous effect on us. Here's how red, green, yellow, blue, and orange affect you and those around you.

RED

Light saver: Dermatologists often treat signs of aging with red LED light treatments, which have been shown to decrease wrinkles and spots. Now you can get similar results at home by using a handheld light-emitting gadget, such as the Tanda Luxe Skin Rejuvenation Device ($195; tanda.com) for 3 minutes, twice a week.

Red alert: Research shows that men rate women wearing this shade as more attractive. Try painting nails with L'Oreal Paris Colour Riche Nail Color in Rendezvous ($6; drugstores).

Berry fit: Smelling strawberries while exercising might burn more calories. Try strawberry-spiked Degree Invisible Solid in Just Dance antiperspirant ($3; drugstores) before workouts.

Real lip service: A greater color contrast between your lips and your skin will make you look more feminine, according to research. A rich scarlet, such as Maybelline New York SuperStay 14HR Lipstick in Ravishing Rouge ($9; drugstores), creates a significant distinction for all skin tones.

To dye for: Red hair dye fades more quickly than other shades because the color molecules are larger, so hair strands have a hard time holding on to them. To prevent red dye—or any color—from washing out, use Redken Color Extend Shampoo ($13.50; redken.com for salons).

Rosy outlook: Sniffing scents with linalool, a compound found in roses, can reduce the activity of stress-activated genes, according to animal research. Next time your nerves are frayed, apply lotion with rose notes, such as Olay Body Lotion in Silk Whimsy ($4; drugstores).

GREEN

Little green giant: Alguronic acid—derived from tiny chlorophyll-rich microalgae—has demonstrated a big anti-aging impact. It's even more effective at boosting elastin production and cell turnover than retinol, according to studies commissioned by Solazyme, a San Francisco biotechnology company. Find it in Algenist Firming & Lifting Intensive Mask ($52; sephora.com).

Super skin brightener: Combat a dull complexion with First Aid Beauty Facial Radiance Pads ($28; firstaidbeauty.com), which contain the skin resurfacer glycolic acid, as well as cucumber. It prevents irritation, so you see glowing skin—not redness.

Hair lifter: Cooling peppermint and refreshing eucalyptus keep your scalp from getting sweaty, so hair doesn't go limp in hot weather. Find them both in John Frieda Root Awakening Lift + Refresh Root Spray ($7; drugstores).

"Green light provides a calming sensation."

Headache helper: Sniffing green apple might ease a migraine. In one study, when people in the midst of a migraine smelled the scent, their pain

SMOOTH MOVES

Facial hair can get coarser and darker with age-related estrogen dips. The following are some safe, effective ways to whisk away those whiskers.

GROWTH-INHIBITING CREAMS: Prescription-only Vaniqa lotion reduces growth but won't remove hair (a 2-month supply costs about $100). For a similar effect, OTC growth-inhibiting creams, such as DermaDoctor Gorilla Warfare Hair Minimizing Facial Moisturizer ($50; ulta.com), slow follicle activity with botanicals such as palmetto and fireweed.

PERMANENT TREATMENTS: Ask your derm about laser hair removal or electrolysis. Each destroys the hair root—with a zap of intense light or an electrical current, respectively.

"Laser removal works by detecting the pigment of the hair, so it's effective only on dark strands," says Anne Chapas, MD, a New York City–based dermatologist. "Electrolysis is good for any hair color." Just watch your pocketbook: Electrolysis can cost $50 and up per session, while laser removal is at least double that. Both treatments require multiple sessions.

DEPILATORY CREAMS: Depilatory creams, such as Nair Precision Face and Upper Lip Kit ($7; drugstores), have a chemical that breaks down the keratin bond in hairs, dissolving them beneath the surface of the skin. Results last about 2 weeks (until the hair grows past the surface again).

WAXING: Salon waxing removes hairs with one swift pull, and you can get the same results at home. Try Sally Hansen Microwaveable Eyebrow, Lip, and Face Wax Kit ($6; drugstores), which doesn't require muslin strips. The wax hardens and you pull it off, along with fuzz.

Mastering sticky waxing can be tricky. But because most facial hair is fine, waxing hurts less here than in other parts of the body. Results last 3 to 6 weeks until a new hair grows.

lessened more than when they weren't smelling anything.

Soothing shades: Green-tinted eyewear, such as Tory Burch sunglasses in Style 6016 ($145; sunglasshut.com), might be better than the proverbial rose-colored glasses. Research suggests that viewing subdued green light enhances the production of dopamine in the brain and provides a calming sensation, says psychologist Richard Wiseman, PhD.

Stimulating scent: Smelling rosemary might help you improve your memory, according to research from the University of Northumbria in the United Kingdom. Find the invigorating note in 21 Drops Focus Aromatherapy Oil Roll-On ($29; 21drops.com).

YELLOW

Flower power: Oil extracted from dandelions can help moisturize hair and soothe a dry, itchy scalp. Find the strand-saving ingredient in Davines NaturalTech Purifying Shampoo ($25; davines.com for salons).

Mega moisture: If you have dry skin, consider taking 360 milligrams of borage seed oil daily. Researchers have found that supplementing with this amount increases the barrier function of skin, decreasing water loss over time. Try Whole Foods Cold Pressed Borage Oil Soft Gels Supplements ($19 for 90; Whole Foods).

Pretty, happy lips: The key to contentment is under your nose when you use Eos Lip Balm SPF 15 Smooth Sphere in Lemon Drop ($3.50; drugstores). The lip protector contains lemon oil—a sniff of which can improve your mood, according to research.

Liquid gold: You can update a nude lipstick by topping it with a golden gloss. "It enhances and adds warmth to the color and reflects light off of lips to make them look plumper," says makeup artist Emily Kate Warren. Try Lancome Juicy Tubes in Touched by Light ($18; lancome-usa.com).

Rise and shine: Start your day off bright with yellow. The sunny hue is associated with happiness and a positive emotional state, according to several studies. For a glowing complexion (and mood!), wash with a yellow Clarisonic Mia Sonic Skin Cleansing System ($119; clarisonic.com).

Fountain of youth: Spray on a grapefruit scent, such as Dove Go Fresh Energizing Body Mist ($4; drugstores), for an instant youth boost. When others smell the zesty scent, they judge you to be up to 5 years younger.

Redness reliever: In a study conducted by the National Rosacea Society, 54 percent of rosacea sufferers said they use yellow-based makeup to offset redness (the shade has a neutralizing effect). If your face flares—whether from rosacea, a sunburn, or sensitivity—dust on Clinique Redness Solutions Instant Relief Mineral Pressed Powder ($32.50; clinique.com), a sheer, yellow-tinted powder with anti-inflammatory caffeine.

Sweet skin saver: Honey—the all-natural kitchen cure for summer skin bummers such as bug bites and scrapes—has been shown to soothe skin and help prevent infection.

BLUE

True blue: Wear this color to make a good impression. It's universally liked, according to research from the UK's University of Manchester, and "it makes you seem trustworthy," says Leslie Harrington, PhD, executive director of the Color Association of the United States.

Try it on eyes: Use your ring finger to swipe a sheer-blue cream shadow, such as Shiseido Shimmering Cream Eye Color in Ice ($25; shiseido.com), along your top lash lines.

Eye opener: Red or bloodshot eyes can make you seem sad, according to research published in *Ethology*. To brighten up, apply a navy mascara, such as Pixi Lash Booster Mascara in Blackest Blue ($17; Target).

"The blue makes the whites of eyes appear whiter," says makeup artist Petra Strand.

Seasonal aroma: Sweet-smelling bluebells burst into bloom in April and May. If you don't live near a wildflower preserve, you can still indulge in the spring-has-arrived scent by stocking your bathroom with a bottle of Mrs. Meyer's Clean Day Bluebell Liquid Hand Soap ($4; mrsmeyers.com).

"Wearing blue makes you seem more trustworthy."

Bruise clues: Snacking on blueberries can help reduce the appearance of any black-and-blue marks. The berries contain flavonoids and vitamin C, which together improve blood circulation to reduce swelling, as well as proanthocyanidins, which help to strengthen the walls of capillaries that are weakened by bruising.

Smooth remover: Prevent irritation when you're taking off stubborn eye makeup by using a cotton pad soaked in a remover that contains cornflower extract, such as Vichy Laboratoires Purete Thermale Eye MakeUp Remover for Sensitive Eyes ($16.50; vichyusa.com). The bright-blue flower contains several anti-inflammatory substances, according to a study in the *Journal of Ethnopharmacology.*

Sun shield: Dark blue clothing offers more protection from UV than colors such as yellow, finds a study in Industrial & Engineering Chemistry Research.

ORANGE

Youth booster: Idebenone is a powerful antioxidant that helps halt signs of aging, like wrinkles, when applied topically. There's also reason to swallow it: The supplement has been shown to improve neurological function in people with Alzheimer's. Try Priori Idebenone Superceuticals Dietary Supplements ($65; prioriskincare.com for locations).

Scalp-friendly spice: Turmeric has been used for hundreds of years as a treatment for hair and scalp issues, according to Dr. Vinod Upadhyay of Maharshi Bhardwaj Clinic and Research Center in Haridwar, India. The antioxidant-rich ingredient is now in 21st-century hair thickeners: the Aveda Invati Collection ($24 and up; aveda.com), a shampoo, conditioner, and treatment spray, which can reduce hair loss by 33 percent in 12 weeks.

The root of good skin: Carrot extract—found in Yes To Carrots Rich Moisture Day Cream ($15; Target)—is a double-duty beautifier for your complexion, providing both moisture for instant benefits and antioxidants that protect skin long-term.

Hand healer: Soften your palms and heal ragged cuticles by applying a dollop of Weleda Sea Buckthorn Hand Cream ($11; usa. weleda.com). It features the lipid-rich oil of bright orange sea buckthorn berries, which are a proven skin hydrator and wound healer.

Hot hue: Pantone teamed with Sephora to create Sephora + Pantone Universe Tangerine Tango Brush Set ($68; sephora.com), a set of five brushes with supersoft bristles in the red-orange hue. They can lend the shade's uplifting, energizing effect to your morning makeup routine without the color commitment of bright orange lipstick.

Suntan snack: For a healthy-looking glow all over, munch on foods high in beta-carotene, such as orange bell peppers. Eating foods high in carotenoids can tint skin slightly over time, and the subtle color change looks better (and is a lot healthier!) than that caused by the sun.

THE ALL-NATURAL EYE LIFT

A touch of liner defines eyes and wakes up your entire face. But as lids lose elasticity and get crepey, it's almost impossible to apply evenly. The following tricks from celebrity makeup artist Mally Roncal, founder of Mally Beauty, help.

Using your finger, blend an eye shadow base, such as Tarte Clean Slate 360 Creaseless Smoothing Eye Primer ($19; ulta.com), all over your lids. It absorbs oils and fills wrinkles, creating a smoother surface for your pencil to skim over.

Line your top lash line using a waterproof pencil with a gel-like consistency, such as Maybelline New York Eye Studio Master Drama Cream Pencil in Bold Brown ($8; drugstores). The formula glides easily but dries quickly, so it won't feather. Pull your lid taut toward your temple and apply the liner inward from the outer corner, wiggling the tip into your lash line as you go. When you release the lid, there won't be any gaps where the color jumped.

Using a chubby eye pencil in a pale, shimmery hue, draw a line directly above the dark-brown liner (with this technique, you can skip shadow). This camouflages uneven texture or messy liner edges, and the shimmer reflects light to brighten areas that might be cast in shadow by heavy lids. Try E.L.F. Studio Waterproof Eyeliner Crayon in Champagne ($3; eyeslipsface.com).

CHAPTER 31

SUN SAFETY

Here's everything you ever wanted to know and were smart enough to ask. Top dermatologists answer all your burning questions about sun protection.

If we lived in pristine, temperature-controlled labs, SPF 15 would be adequate—if not optimal—protection against sunburn (caused by UVB rays) and skin aging and cancer (caused by UVA and UVB rays). But we live in the real (sweaty, splashy, windy) world, and we don't use as much sunscreen as we should.

In fact, the protection most of us get from SPF 15 is more like SPF 3 to 7. That's why the American Academy of Dermatology recommends using broad-spectrum SPF 30. It's great advice, but it doesn't clear up all the sun-safety confusion. So we asked the experts to solve your toughest quandaries, one by one.

What's the highest SPF that's legit? I heard it's 50. So why do I see products with much higher numbers? If you apply sunscreen correctly (see "Sunscreen Rules" on page 347), SPF 50 offers the maximum protection necessary.

You're seeing SPF 80 and even SPF 110 on shelves because of "marketing, marketing, marketing," says Bruce Katz, MD, a dermatologist in New York City. Companies know that higher numbers make you think you're getting a significant surplus of protection, even though you're not. But the FDA has caught on to this strategy and proposed a rule making "50+" the highest SPF value allowed. The rule hasn't been approved yet, but many manufacturers are probably betting it will. They're already distributing products labeled SPF 50+, even as they continue to sell higher numbers.

Are sun-protective hair products a waste of money? The sun can change your hair color, but products with UV filters or antioxidants might keep your hue from fading or turning brassy. If you like the color you've got (or spent good money to get), a spray such as Paul Mitchell Sun Shield Conditioning Spray ($18; paulmitchell.com for salons) helps.

Will it prevent cancer? No, and cancer commonly forms on the scalp, says Dr. Katz. You should still wear a hat or use traditional SPF on your part—or your entire scalp if your hair is thin.

I hate it when I'm outdoors or exercising and my eyes start stinging from drippy sunscreen. What are my options? That burning is usually caused by chemical sunscreens (ingredients listed on the Drug Facts label that end with "-ate," "-ene," or "-one," such as homosalate, octocrylene, or oxybenzone). Instead, look for a water-resistant product with physical (sometimes called mineral or natural) sunscreen, such as zinc oxide or titanium dioxide. Even with those guidelines, it can take time to find the right formula, because fragrance can also sting. We tried a few dozen, and the clear-eyed winner was—MDSolarSciences Natural Mineral Sunscreen Stick SPF 40 ($13; mdsolarsciences.com).

How long does the SPF in my moisturizer last? If you don't plan to work up a sweat or be outside long, the protection should last 2 to 4 hours, says Amy

ANTI-AGING FOR THE ABSENTMINDED

Use a lotion with antioxidants for 2 weeks, and you could continue to get UV–protection benefits for 3 additional days—even if you don't reapply the lotion, according to new research.

Wechsler, MD, a dermatologist in New York City. But if you'll be outdoors, you need a water-resistant sunscreen in addition to (or instead of) your usual moisturizer. L'Oreal Paris Sublime Sun Liquid Silk Sunshield for Face SPF 50+ ($11; drugstores) is as lightweight as a face lotion.

Any advice for applying sunscreen to your own back? Reaching up and over your shoulder, you should be able to get the job done with a clear, continuous spray that works upside down. Aveeno's HydroSport Sunblock Spray SPF 30 ($10; drugstores) propels about 2 feet and should reach even the center of your back. If you're not flexible enough for the reach-over, slip on a tank top with UPF (ultraviolet protection factor). You can make your own by washing a top you like in SunGuard ($2; sunguardsunprotection.com). It coats clothing with an undetectable layer of UPF 30 that lasts up to 20 washes.

I was diagnosed with a basal cell carcinoma, and it was removed. My doctor says I have to be even more careful about sun protection. Why? Skin cancer survivors are much more likely to develop a second skin cancer, says Erin Gilbert, MD, PhD, a dermatologist in New York City. That's because they've already accumulated enough UV harm near the original cancer (derms call it field damage) to make getting another likely. For survivors, skin exams every 6 months are essential. Everyone else should get one yearly—sooner if you have a suspicious mole.

I've been trying to eat healthier, and as my diet gets cleaner, I seem to burn less. Why would that be? Certain nutrients, especially phytochemicals, improve skin's ability to ward off damage. One study found that supplementing with lycopene (a pigment found in red fruits and vegetables) might prevent UV damage; another showed that people taking a supplement with alpha- and beta-carotenoids (in orange and yellow produce) were less likely to have skin damage after UV exposure. It's possible that eating a rainbow could delay sunburn, but that doesn't mean a salad is equal to sunscreen.

Is sunscreen residue bad for marine life? Yes. Some ingredients in sunscreen can awaken viruses that kill coral's food supply—and ultimately, the reefs themselves and the animals that live there. The common ingredients that are most damaging include oxybenzone and the preservative butylparaben.

For an eco-friendly option, choose a product that uses the physical sunscreen ingredients zinc oxide or titanium dioxide because they "break down more readily in nature," says Ni'Kita Wilson, a cosmetic chemist in New Jersey.

I have rosacea. Should I be using regular sunscreen on my face, or do I need something special? Rosacea makes skin sensitive and more likely to react to certain ingredients in sunscreen, but the sun itself is one of the biggest flare-up triggers, so going unprotected is not an option.

Robin Schaffran, MD, a dermatologist in Los Angeles, suggests avoiding chemical sunscreens, and Dr. Wechsler also tells her patients with rosacea to say no to fragrance. Neutrogena Pure & Free Liquid Daily Sunblock SPF 50 ($14; drugstores) is a good option. Or try Colorescience Sunforgettable Face Primer SPF 30 ($50; colorescience.com), which has a tint that helps hide redness.

Can you recommend a natural sunscreen that doesn't look like toothpaste? The purest options are those without chemical sunscreens, retinyl palmitate, fragrance, or parabens. That leaves products that use physical sunscreens, which typically don't rub in as easily and sometimes leave skin with a whitish cast. After trying pretty much every natural sunscreen that meets these guide-lines (for a list, go to prevention.com/natural sunscreen), we found the least toothpasty, most pleasing picks were Banana Boat Natural Reflect SPF 50+ ($11.50; drugstores) and All Terrain TerraSport SPF 30 Spray ($14; allterrainco .com).

Is there any reason to wear sun-protective clothing? The best sun defense isn't sunscreen alone, so wearing cover-ups can help. But white cotton has only about UPF 5 to 7, and colored cotton has about UPF 10. Black velvet or dark denim can have up to UPF 50, but who wants to wear denim—not to mention velvet!—all summer? Instead, look for UPF 30 sweat-wicking clothes. Try columbia.com.

I know too much sun can cause cancer, but aren't the chemicals in sunscreens unhealthy too? Although a few studies have raised questions about the safety of two ingredients in some sunscreens, you can find products without them if you're worried.

Oxybenzone has been shown to cause hormone disruption in cancer cells,

SUNSCREEN YOU CAN SWALLOW?

Even if it's the middle of winter and your shorts and swimsuits are packed away, that doesn't mean you're safe from the sun. UVA radiation, which causes aging and skin damage that can lead to cancer, remains at almost the same intensity year-round.

"Even if you're not turning red, your skin can be damaged," says holistic dermatologist Alan M. Dattner, MD. Sun-protective clothing and sunscreen are two ways to ensure you're protected, but some herbs, when taken orally, might boost your skin's ability to protect against UV rays, research shows.

GREEN TEA: Every leaf is chock-full of EGCG, an antioxidant that can decrease sun damage when applied topically. But drinking green tea might protect skin as well, says Dr. Dattner. One study showed that drinking 3 cups of green tea a day increases the ability of blood cells to protect themselves against damage caused by UV exposure, and it's possible that skin cells might also benefit from green-tea protection.

FRENCH MARITIME PINE BARK: Taking a supplement of the extract of this tree (sold as Pycnogenol) has been shown to inhibit inflammation caused by UV exposure and protect against sunburns.

POLYPODIUM LEUCOTOMOS: The extract of this antioxidant-rich fern—also known by its Spanish name, calaguala—has been shown to raise the threshold of sun exposure that the body can take without burning. Find it in Heliocare ($32; drugstore.com); a capsule a day is the suggested dose.

but a study of its effect on skin showed no statistically significant changes. Large doses of retinyl palmitate have been linked to skin cancer in mice that are susceptible to the disease, but no human studies show that it causes cancer, says Steven Q. Wang, director of dermatology for Memorial Sloan-Kettering Cancer Center in Basking Ridge, New Jersey.

Are sport sunscreens really waterproof? First, ignore the word "sport" on labels. It might imply some sort of water or sweat resistance, but the government doesn't regulate the use of the term, so you can't be sure.

What you can be sure of is this: "No sunscreen is truly waterproof or sweat-proof," says Dr. Katz. That's why in June 2011, the FDA passed a rule banning the use of the terms waterproof and sweatproof. Soon the most water- and sweat-resistant sunscreen you can get will be labeled "water-resistant (80 minutes)," such as Coppertone Sport Pro Series SPF 50+ ($11; drugstores).

SUNSCREEN STATS

Here are some simple sunscreen rules, by the numbers.

SUNSCREEN RULE #1

30 The minimum SPF you should use. Other must-haves are water resistance and a broad-spectrum formula.

SUNSCREEN RULE #2

20 The number of minutes before you go out in the sun that you should apply sunscreen. You can skip this rule if your lotion has titanium dioxide or zinc oxide, which are effective immediately.

SUNSCREEN RULE #3

1 OUNCE The amount of sunscreen you should use to coat your body with enough product (a 0.002 mm layer) to provide the SPF listed on the label. If you're using lotion, that's about the amount that would fill a shot glass. If you're using a clear, continuous spray, that's 30 to 90 seconds of spraying—enough to create a visibly glossy sheen as it goes on.

SUNSCREEN RULE #4

2 The number of hours you can go without reapplying if you're not sweating or in the water.

SUNSCREEN RULE #5

40 PERCENT That's how much less likely people who regularly take vitamin A supplements are to develop melanoma, compared with those who don't. The possible reason is that vitamin A might stop the cancer cells from multiplying.

LOVIN' LIFE

The delightful Jamie Lee Curtis talks about finding courage, her love of books, and the joy of life on the other side of 50.

"A woman I admire a lot said to me, 'God makes you age to show you that you don't have time to waste,'" says Jamie Lee Curtis, 55. "It really stuck with me. It's the reason I look for meaning in my life, my relationships, and my friendships."

Such deliberate focus takes courage. That's one reason Curtis has made it the theme of her 10th book for children, *My Brave Year of Firsts: Tries, Sighs, and High Fives*, which celebrates the everyday daring of trying new things from the perspective of a 6-year-old girl named Frankie. It's a powerful notion for Curtis.

"Humans are so brave," she says, "especially in a modern world with working parents who are trying so hard to keep it all going. But women are particularly brave, probably because we're the caretakers."

Ever amiable, Curtis was happy to sit down for a candid conversation about the satisfaction of writing a new book and the gratitude she feels for her life.

Prevention: It seems like you're loving life on the other side of 50.

Curtis: You see the consequences of the choices you've made. You develop a real point of view, and hopefully, you use all that knowledge to make some impact in the lives of your children and family, which ripples out in concentric circles.

Prevention: What's your next "first"?

Curtis: I actually don't know. I've never been someone who plans anything. A little part of me leaves my body and goes, How did you land this life, this house, those dogs, that husband, those kids, that work? Honestly, every good thing that's happened to me took place when I didn't know it was going to. Everything I've tried to control and manipulate has worked, but it hasn't been transformative. My experience has taught me to keep the channels open and get rid of obstacles—first by accepting that they exist and then by doing something about them.

Prevention: Can you share an example from your own life?

Curtis: Yes. I got sober. I had understood for a long time that my relationship with drugs and alcohol was a problem. But because I was successful in so many

JAMIE'S BEST-LOVED BOOKS

Avid reader (and writer) Jamie Lee Curtis shared her all-time favorite books with us.

EAST OF EDEN, by John Steinbeck: The biblical account of Cain and Abel is reflected through the lens of one family.

THE TRANSIT OF VENUS, by Shirley Hazzard: This intricate novel follows two sisters starting a new life after World War II.

SHOGUN, by James Clavell: A tale of a bold English adventurer embroiled in the feudal politics of a war-torn Japan.

ANGLE OF REPOSE, by Wallace Stegner: A Pulitzer Prize–winning chronicle of four generations of an American family.

GO, DOG. GO, by P. D. Eastman: A kids' classic since 1961.

ways, it disguised itself as recreation and fun. Still, I had a gnawing awareness that there was something bigger at play. So my awareness and then acceptance of the problem was a very big deal for me. I'm very lucky that I've been sober for almost 14 years.

Prevention: Another recent first for you was running the Santa Monica Classic, a 5-K.

Curtis: I ran that race to face my fear. Everywhere I go, people say to me, "You're great. I love you." Somehow all of that felt fraudulent in that I couldn't run a mile. The longer you avoid a fear, it just grows.

Prevention: Did you have a trainer?

Curtis: Nope. I prepared for it by myself, and I ran it by myself. To train, I used an iPhone app called Couch-to-5K. I cried at the finish line. That 5-K was a big deal for me.

Prevention: What other "first" would you love to try?

Curtis: If there was a 100 percent guarantee that I wouldn't get hurt, I'd jump out of a plane in a heartbeat. I'd be the first person at the airfield.

Prevention: You and your husband, Christopher Guest, have two kids: Annie, who's 27, and Tom, 17. Now that they're older, are you starting to explore different ways to spend time with each other?

Curtis: We play golf together. That's been a first. My husband calls me the Hammer because I can hit a golf ball pretty far. We've been home together for a considerable amount of time, which has been lovely. We've fallen into the pleasure of simultaneous reading.

> "Honestly, every good thing that's happened to me took place when I didn't know it was going to."

Prevention: What have you read lately?

Curtis: Two summers ago, my sister and I went to Germany, Denmark, and Hungary. When I travel, I like to read one piece of fiction and one of nonfiction that are set in the place I'm headed. So when I get there, I can go, Oh, yeah. I read a harrowing book set in Hungary in the Second World War, called *The Invisible Bridge,* and Wallace Stegner's *The Spectator Bird,* a lovely story that takes place in Denmark.

Prevention: There have been some great movie roles for women lately, like those in *Hope Springs* and *The Best Exotic Marigold Hotel.* Do you think it's a trend?

Curtis: Obviously, there's a huge audience dying for entertainment that they can relate to, and it's not *Transformers.*

Prevention: One of our favorite moments in your book is when Frankie jumps off the cliff into a lake. What was your first metaphorical jump?

Curtis: For me, the leap was and is to stay out of our kids' way so that they have their chance to jump and not be tethered to you. Parenting is so hard because it's the only time in your life when the goal of a relationship is separation.

Prevention: Does it take courage to make new friends when you are an adult?

"Parenting is so hard because it's the only time in your life when the goal of a relationship is separation."

Curtis: I make friends very easily everywhere I go. If we get in an elevator, my family will look at me and go, "Please don't. Please." It's just my nature. With real friends, people whom I get intimate with, it's harder. I've had a beautiful opening of wonderful new friendships in my life in the past 10 years. I don't have the patience for trivial friendships anymore. I can't hear the same complaints about the ex-husband. It's heartbreaking to me to think that we can't learn from our developmental mistakes and then grow.

Prevention: You've been very adept at discovering your true voice. Why do you think it's easier for some women than others?

Curtis: For me, writing books has allowed me to have a voice. Everyone has ideas. They just don't often have a place to put them. No matter what, writing what's in your head is a very good thing to do. Whether or not it's going to get published or it lives on a blog, there's more and more availability for expression. And that's really great.

"Everyone has ideas. They just don't often have a place to put them."

PHOTO CREDITS

INDEX

Underscored page references indicate boxed text and tables.
Boldface references indicate photographs and illustrations.

Processed foods
    prebiotics in, 214
    probiotics in, 212
    reducing in diet, 200, 218
    sugar content of, 94
Produce. *See* Fruit; Vegetables
Profiles. *See Prevention* profiles
Protein
    for bone health, 24
    including in diet, 195
    muscle loss and, 74
    recommended intake of, 197
    to reduce belly fat, 149, 153, 156
    vegetable sources, 7
Pumpkin-Bacon Pancakes, 123
Pumpkin seeds, 123
Pure Fruit Pigmented Lip and Cheek
        Tint, 318
Puristics Totally Ageless products, 302
Purple produce, 301
Push-ups
    Chaturanga, 107, **107**
    inchworm with, 162, **162**
    in walking workout, 168, **168**

Q

Qigong, 40
Quadruped balance, 157, 157
Quercetin, 303
Quizzes
    bad habits, 261
    food safety, 13, 14
    hair type, 325

R

Rainbow diet, 7
Raspberries
    Pistachio Clouds with Fresh Fruit, 130

Reading, Jamie Lee Curtis on, 350,
        351–52
Rear deltoid fly (suspension strap), 141,
        141
Recipes
    Asparagus and Chicken Fricassee, 202
    Baked Maple Pears, 131
    Grilled Chicken with Mango Mojo, 127
    Grilled Vegetable Pasta Salad, 125
    Mango-Shrimp Rice Noodles, 129
    Mushroom Pizzas, 126
    Pear Toddy, 122
    Pistachio Clouds with Fresh Fruit, 130
    Pumpkin-Bacon Pancakes, 123
    Roasted Zucchini No-Noodle Lasagna,
        205
    Sausage-Stuffed Mushrooms, 124
    Sea Scallop Surf & Turf, 206
    Steak, Peppers, and Mashed Potatoes,
        128
    Tuscan Spinach Dumplings with
        White Beans, 203
    Very Veggie Pasta Toss, 204
Red Bull, 49
Red color therapy, 333–34
Redken Body Full Shampoo, 325
Redkin Color Extend Shampoo, 334
Reebok Urlead, 176
Refrigerators, food safety and, 13
REI Traverse Shocklight Women's
        Trekking Poles, 182
Religion, Goldie Hawn on, 290–91
Republic of Tea Iced Tea, The, 86
Restrictive sleep therapy, 284
Resveratrol, 317
Reverse crunch, 154, **154**
Reverse Warrior to Side Angle, 105, **105**
Rice alternative, 196–97
Rimmel London Volume Accelerator
        Mascara, 319–20